ROUTLEDGE LIBRARY EDITIONS: AGING

Volume 2

DAY BROUGHT BACK MY NIGHT

DAY BROUGHT BACK MY NIGHT

Aging and New Vision Loss

STEPHEN CHARLES AINLAY

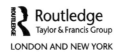

Routledge
Taylor & Francis Group

LONDON AND NEW YORK

First published in 1989 by Routledge

This edition first published in 2024
by Routledge
4 Park Square, Milton Park, Abingdon, Oxon OX14 4RN

and by Routledge
605 Third Avenue, New York, NY 10158

Routledge is an imprint of the Taylor & Francis Group, an informa business

British Library Cataloguing in Publication Data
A catalogue record for this book is available from the British Library

ISBN: 978-1-032-67433-9 (Set)
ISBN: 978-1-032-67928-0 (Volume 2) (hbk)
ISBN: 978-1-032-67943-3 (Volume 2) (pbk)
ISBN: 978-1-032-67941-9 (Volume 2) (ebk)

DOI: 10.4324/9781032679419

Publisher's Note
The publisher has gone to great lengths to ensure the quality of this reprint but points out that some imperfections in the original copies may be apparent.

Disclaimer
The publisher has made every effort to trace copyright holders and would welcome correspondence from those they have been unable to trace.

DAY BROUGHT BACK MY NIGHT

Aging and New Vision Loss

Stephen Charles Ainlay

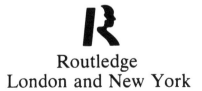

Routledge
London and New York

First published in 1989
by Routledge
11 New Fetter Lane, London EC4P 4EE
29 West 35th Street, New York, NY 10001

© 1989 Stephen Charles Ainlay

Typeset by Photoprint, Torquay, Devon
Printed and bound in Great Britain by
Mackays of Chatham PLC, Chatham, Kent

British Library Cataloguing in Publication Data

Ainlay, Stephen C. (Stephen Charles), *1951*–
Day brought back my night.
1. Old persons. Sight disorders.
Psychological aspects
I. Title
618.97'77'0019
ISBN 0–415–00764–X

Library of Congress Cataloging in Publication Data

Ainlay, Stephen C., 1951–
   Day brought back my night : aging and new vision loss / Stephen
Charles Ainlay
      p. cm.
   Bibliography: p.
   Includes index.
   1. Aged, Blind – United States. 2. Blindness – United States –
Psychological aspects. I. Title.
HV1597.5.A35 1989
362.4'1'0880565 – dc 19   88–18288
                                                                      CIP

ISBN 0–415–00764–X

To the Memory of Steven Kent Massanari
1951–1981

Contents

Preface

Darkness. It is one of the most common metaphors used to describe the world of blindness. Most people commonly assume that to be blind is to be in a world of perpetual darkness, and the terror of darkness carries over to the fear most have of the loss of sight. Literature has capitalized on and fed these assumptions and fears, often arguing the similarities between blindness and the darkness of the tomb. Biblical imagery has stressed the links between darkness and blindness *per se*, as well as darkness and an empty life, darkness and evil. The personal anguish of blind Oedipus and his horror at a life of impenetrable darkness, or Samson's despair at his blindness, are also typical of the handling of the imagery in literature. In both literature and common sense we have often associated light with knowledge and goodness, whereas darkness has been associated with ignorance and evil.

Ironically, darkness may be one of the least appropriate descriptions of the experience of blindness – at least in terms of the actual physiological experience. Few people who are counted as 'blind' actually experience darkness. In the first place, only a small fraction have no remaining light perception. Secondly, those who are 'totally blind' seldom report that their experience of blindness is that of being in darkness.

This book explores age-related vision loss. Over two-thirds of all persons who experience severe vision loss in the United States are over age 65. About half of those who have been designated as 'legally blind' are also over 65 (a figure that is suspected to greatly underestimate the prevalence of blindness in later life). Most of these people experience the loss of sight as part of the aging process. Cataracts, glaucoma, macular degeneration, and other age-related disorders slowly deteriorate their visual sensory skills. The loss is so slow in most cases that persons experiencing vision loss in late life will not live long enough to lose all their sight. For them, critical light and color perception, as well as the ability to discern some movement, remain part of their visual experience. Again, the darkness imagery seems somewhat ill-suited to describing their experience.

Given the inappropriateness of the darkness metaphor, one might justifiably question the reasons for titling this volume *Day Brought Back My Night*. Does this risk perpetuating misconceptions of the blind and their experience? I suppose for those who don't read the book there is such a risk; as Michael Monbeck (1973: 6) has pointed out, other point guards in the effort to change people's views about blindness have ended up only reinforcing negative stereotypes. Publications for persons experiencing blindness, with titles like *Lookout, Beacon, Outlook*, may have quite unintentionally perpetuated notions that blindness necessarily brings with it gloom, fear, loneliness, and 'whatever the timorous seeing experience in the dark' (Cutsforth, quoted in Monbeck 1973). Will the title to this book do likewise?

I hope not, and don't believe that it will. In fact, I have selected this title quite self-consciously for a number of reasons. To begin with, it provides a foil by which I can address the rather simple yet fundamental insight that it *is* a misconception – a misconception generated and perpetuated by a sighted world that has systematically avoided the world of blindness and segregated those who experience it from the mainstream of life.

I have decided to use this title for a second reason as well. Since most persons who are blind and severely visually impaired have spent their lives as sighted persons, they share many of the same misconceptions of blindness, and carry them into their own experience of vision loss. They often have intense fears of blindness, precisely because they too associate it with darkness, ignorance, evil, along with helplessness. Correspondingly, to understand their fears and their struggles it is important to understand the significance of the darkness imagery. When asked what they fear most, many persons who have lost sight (to the point of qualifying as legally blind or severely visually impaired) will tell you that it is the darkness of total blindness that keeps them awake and spawns much of their anguish. Assurances that it will never happen – whether these come from medical professionals, services providers, family, or friends – do little to quell their fears.

The title of this book takes its inspiration from John Milton's Sonnet XXIII ('Methought I saw my late espoused saint,' 1969). Milton was well familiar with tragedy. His first wife died in 1652 when he was in his early forties. He married again four years later. His second wife died short of her thirtieth birthday after they had been married just two years. The daughter Milton had by his second marriage died six weeks after her mother. Sonnet XXIII betrays some of the pain left by these experiences. It specifically aims to be an expression of Milton's sentiments for his second wife. He uses the vehicle of a dream – in which she comes and goes – to speak of his feelings for her. It captures, however, the tragedy not simply of her death and the death of their child, but also of the despair that can accompany the loss of sight. Milton had lost his sight at about the time of the death of his first wife, and the impact of the loss is evident at various places in his writing. For example, he never saw his second wife. Hence, in Sonnet XXIII, he speaks of her face veiled to even his fancied sight. He also speaks of the promise of seeing her that heaven holds. Perhaps more notably, it speaks of his ongoing experience of blindness as well when, at the end, he indicates that upon awakening 'day brought back my night.'

While never handled so succinctly as in the final words of this sonnet, Milton addressed his reactions to blindness in other works as well. Sonnet XIX ('When I consider how my light is spent') is a more self-conscious response to the loss of sight, and the agony of his blindness in Samson Agonistes seems transparently auto-biographical. In the case of the former he speaks of his days in 'this dark world.' In the latter, the chorus speaks of Samson's blindness as 'prison within prison inseparably dark' – again the darkness metaphor used to capture blindness. But here it is used by a person experiencing vision loss to capture not so much the physiological experience but, as metaphors are intended to do, the sighted person's dread of the condition.

Milton affords a poetic glimpse at the fear, frustration, and sometime despair that nearly all persons who lose their sight confront at one time or another. These are important aspects of the experience of blindness and they are a critical part of the story of aging and vision loss. This is not to say, however, that the story ends here. As will be seen in the chapters to follow, many people come to terms with their vision loss and the fears, frustrations, and despair recede into the background of the business of living. Nevertheless, the use of the darkness imagery forces us to come to terms with this tension in the experience of blindness. We cannot simply dismiss sighted persons' misconceptions of blindness as wrong, because these same misconceptions inform the perspective of those who lose sight in late life. Overcoming such misconceptions may prove one of the most challenging and difficult tasks that the older person facing vision loss will confront.

This book is also a study of identity; how people maintain a sense of themselves as having continuity – continuity of situation, continuity of character. I will argue that it is fruitless to speak of identity without examining human aging. Maintaining identity means coming to terms with changing biological and social contexts. Aging (the process of growing up and growing old) poses, by definition, the problem of identity maintenance; that is, coming to terms with a changing body and a changing social environment is part and parcel of the aging process. Some changes are so minor as to be unnoticeable. Others are quite dramatic. In any case, just as aging is inherent in issues of identity, change – physiological and social – is equally inherent in human aging. The unity of identity, aging, and processual change through the course of life will become apparent as we study age-related vision loss. Such changes are not, of course, restricted to later life. Puberty, for example, forces a substantial overhaul of the adolescent's sense of situation and character, just as does blindness in late life. This is true not only because each life event poses equally substantial physiological changes, but also because they carry with them major changes in both relationships with others and the institutions in which life is carried on.

There is a third reason for deciding to use the title that I have for this book. Sociologists have sometimes discussed such major life changes under the rubric of what they term 'anomy' – that is, they argue that dramatic changes threaten meaninglessness. How do people make sense of themselves and their worlds in the face of these changes? What happens if they can't make sense of them? The use of the title metaphor with regard to vision loss is again appropriate with regard to identity because 'darkness' has also been used to describe the 'lurking irrealities' that are part of life experience. As Peter Berger has put it, 'every socially constructed nomos must face the constant possibility of its collapse into anomy' and, invoking the imagery of darkness, 'seen in the perspective of the individual, every nomos represents the bright "dayside" of life, tenuously held onto against the sinister shadows of the "night"' (1967: 23).

Vision loss poses one such lurking irreality, and as such threatens the shadows of anomy. But it is by no means unique. All of us face, in our own respective ways, different threats to our *nomos* – our meaningful ordering of experience. Each of us must contend with our own shadows. Likewise, all of us must struggle to restore meaning when it is threatened. Thought of in these terms, the title of this book could be applied to the study of any event, situation, or circumstance that raises the specter of anomy. As such, vision loss will be used to give us insight, some understanding of a basic human problem: Where and how do we find meaning for our lives and for ourselves? The story that will be told here will tell as much about the essential human struggle to maintain an ordered sense of self and world – of reality – as it does about the experiential idiosyncrasies of losing one's sight.

Acknowledgements

The completion of the study would not have been possible without the postdoctoral support of the Rutgers/Princeton Program in Mental Health Studies (National Institute for Mental Health grant number MH 16242). Similarly a Batchelor (Ford) Faculty Fellowship from Holy Cross College, as well as a grant from its Committee on Research and Publications, were critical to final manuscript preparation.

There are numerous people who helped facilitate this study. To single them out is to risk omitting others. Nevertheless, a special debt is owed to the people who offered advice and support. Peter Berger, Robert Scott, Anne Foner, D. Randall Smith, John Ainlay, Gaylene Becker, Donald Redfoot, James Hunter, Edward Rhine, Paul Collins, Victoria Swigert, Mark Freeman, Suzanne Keller, Gail Filion, Corinne Kirchner, Steven Massanari among others offered comments on early drafts and/or proved reliable sounding boards. Each of them shared her/his insights on various problem areas that are addressed in the book. I would also like to thank the people who reviewed the book for Routledge. The manuscript is undoubtedly better for the comments they made. I am also grateful to Chris Rojek, senior editor in sociology at Routledge, for his advice and handling of the manuscript. And I owe my thanks to Ann Papagni who was very helpful in preparing the manuscript.

A special acknowledgement is owed to Judy Gardner Ainlay who tolerated the numerous 'problematics' that this project posed to our own daily lives and whose work with the elderly provided me with checks on the accuracy of my contentions regarding the experience of late life. I would also be remiss not to acknowledge that my children – Jess and Jonathan – had to bear with me on this project and I thank them for their patience. Charles and Dorothy Ainlay found themselves involved in ways I'm sure they could never have anticipated, from helping with key equipment to assist-

Acknowledgements

ing in transcribing the interviews. In fact, my entire 'extended' family was supportive in so many different ways.

Finally, I must extend my heartfelt thanks to the people who participated in the life history interviews which are central to the study. Without their willingness to share their experiences with me, this study could truly not have been completed. I cannot thank them enough for giving me the time and the patience I required to capture their stories.

Chapter one

Aging and vision loss

Most studies of human aging these days begin with the near-obligatory observation that the elderly in contemporary society constitute an increasing portion of the total population. The population age 65 and older in the United States grew from about 4 per cent of the total population (about 3 million persons) in 1900 to almost 11 per cent of the population (about 25 million) in 1980. If we are to believe the Census Bureau's projections for the future, by the year 2000 persons over 65 will constitute over 12 per cent of the total population (about 32 million persons) and growth will continue into the next century. This ubiquitous observation is not so much a function of authors' redundancies but is rather more a consequence of the profound implications this demographic change has for the age structure of our society, the extent of age-related problems it will carry with it, and the policy planning it necessitates. What are the special needs of an aging population? What implications will this have for social security? How will health-care facilities have to change? The demographic realities of the 'graying of America' have prompted these and other questions. It has also given rise to increased numbers of service professionals who specialize in programs for the elderly, spawned research on aging, and prompted a multitude of gerontology courses on college and university campuses nationwide. These developments have, in turn, raised people's consciousness about the elderly and, indeed, their own aging.

This book aims to continue the process of consciousness raising. It continues this process by drawing attention to a particular age-related health problem. It is an inquiry into sighted people's encounter with the loss of vision in late life. More specifically, it is concerned with how people who confront severe sensory loss maintain a sense of sameness and continuity – a sense of identity. As such the study is concerned with much more than the physiology of vision loss. It unravels the story of older people's

1

confrontations with their changing bodies and social world as well as their personal struggle to provide meaning to these changes when such meaning is not always readily apparent. It is a story of crisis and courage, fear and despair, lost plans and new initiatives. It is a story of a heretofore largely neglected population whose experiences tell much about the life drama that all of us face.

Howard Stewart: a case in point

Howard had celebrated his 67th birthday just four months earlier. All but the oldest of his children had come by the house for dinner and appropriate festivities. Now he and his wife, Estelle, were on their way to visit that oldest son and his family in Pennsylvania. Estelle had been driving the past two hours and as they approached the Philadelphia suburbs the traffic became heavy, the exit signs more frequent. Howard, hoping to fulfill his role as navigator, began looking for the Jenkintown exit. The signs were the green sort that adorn most interstates these days. Several years earlier, Howard had read the same type of sign to minimize the boredom of long trips such as this. To Howard's dismay, however, today he and Estelle would pass the signs before he was able to make out any of the words. He commented, almost casually, that he would have to schedule the appointment with his optometrist that he had been putting off for some time.

The Stewarts' son, Bill, voiced his endorsement of the plan to consult the optometrist. He told his father – half jokingly, half seriously – that the time had come to start taking better care of himself. Although Bill was only just getting used to the idea that his father was retired, he had managed to appoint himself as the offspring most responsible for seeing that his parents were looked after in the later years of life. As if to document the potential improvements that new glasses would make, Bill produced a magnifying glass and the morning newspaper. Yes, maybe new glasses would do the trick.

Howard had been wearing glasses since his early 30s. He had found them annoying at first, but came to accept them as symptomatic of people 'his age.' Several times before he had put off going to the optometrist until he noticed difficulties in reading the newspaper, magazines, and the like. He had no reason to believe that this time would be any different. Since some time around his 40th birthday, his optometrist – a Dr Lewis – had been insisting that he have glaucoma tests. True, the small puff of air in the eye that was involved in the new test was less troublesome than the older method, but it was not something Howard relished.

More than this, however, there was the wait that seemed to face him whenever he had to visit doctors of any sort, and the optometrist was no exception. Making people wait this way seemed antithetical to everything Howard had learned during his years in business.

Howard recounted the trip to Philadelphia to Dr Lewis. Lewis saw many people who were close to Howard Stewart's age. He often listened patiently to their complaints about the long wait to see him and the ineffectiveness of his eyeglass prescriptions. He sometimes thought to himself that life would be easier if he restricted his practice to younger patients. His examination of Howard Stewart, however, signaled problems that he knew extended beyond his professional purview. It seemed to Howard that Dr Lewis was being somewhat evasive. He was certainly not making himself clear as to the nature of Howard's visual difficulties.

Somewhat baffled by the disciplinary boundaries that separated them, Howard nevertheless followed his optometrist's instructions and arranged for an appointment with a local ophthalmologist. Howard had little doubt as to the thoroughness of the examination, given the various gadgets that were used and the many pictures that were taken. When Howard returned two weeks later, the ophthalmologist spoke of the eye as being something like a camera. He talked about visual images, lens, and pointed to a model of the human eye. All of this information became lost, however, to a much more technical phrase, 'macular degeneration' – a condition that was robbing Howard Stewart of his clear central vision.

Almost more perplexing than the impenetrable jargon that always seemed to be involved in the ophthalmologist's answers to Howard's questions was the all-too-clear message he was receiving about the medical remedies that were available. 'I'm afraid there's not much we can do to correct the problem.' Strangely enough, Howard thought about the Apollo flight to the moon that he had believed would never come in his lifetime, and then turned the words 'there is nothing that we can do' over in his mind. All the while the ophthalmologist was reporting the wonderful advances that had been made in low-vision aids – sophisticated magnifying glasses, telescopic lenses, closed-circuit televisions. To say that Howard was even half listening to this discussion would have been generous.

On a subsequent visit, the phrase that really paralyzed Howard emerged. 'You're legally blind.' Howard experienced an array of images – Patty Duke, as Helen Keller groping at the pump mouthing something that resembled the word 'water,' and Jim Carlisle, a World War II vet who used to go door-to-door selling cheap Christmas cards, were two of the most vivid.

Partly out of frustration, partly out of disbelief, Howard sought out the opinion of a second ophthalmologist who practiced in a nearby, but significantly larger, city. His diagnosis only confirmed what the other doctor had told him. Again the discussion of the eye as a camera, again the model, and again the phrases 'There's nothing we can do,' 'You're legally blind.' This time around, Howard sought answers to some questions that had been plaguing him. Would his sight get worse? Hard to say, but likely. How fast would it progress? Hard to say, but more than likely it would occur slowly. Would he go blind – 'really' blind, not this legal blindness? Not likely (the doctor knew that Howard Stewart would probably die before he lost all his remaining vision).

Despite the answers to his questions, Howard returned home after this second visit with a greater sense of helplessness than he had had after the first ophthalmological exam. He searched his memory for something he had done that might have prompted the condition. He asked himself: How could he continue to do the things he enjoyed? What would become of the retirement plans that he and Estelle had been making for ten years now? How much worse would his eyesight become? Suppose the doctor was wrong, suppose he really went blind – what then? In Howard's view, the deterioration of his sight already experienced and that which he felt sure was yet to come meant that his life was over.

In fact, the struggle was just beginning.

Accessing the experience of age-related vision loss

Howard Stewart is fictitious in name only. His experiences are far from unique. While the specific etiology of his condition varies from others' experiences of vision loss, as does the circumstance of his first awareness of the loss of sight, his initial trials with medical professionals, his thoughts and frustration, are typical. So too will be many of the struggles he and others like him face; the struggles with self doubt, the struggles with service providers and medical professionals, the struggles with family and friends – these will be all too typical. It is the intent of this study to detail this typicality by presenting the experiences of older persons who have actually experienced the severe loss of sight – not only the initial experience, but also the subsequent impact of the loss on their sense of their bodies, their physical environment, and their social world.

Older persons who experience blindness or visual impairment carry a double burden. We ignore their blindness because of the uneasiness we have about the condition. We further ignore them because they are old, 'past their prime,' and services geared specifically to them are not viewed as cost effective. Ironically, the elderly constitute the largest segment of the total population of persons with blindness and yet have received the least amount of attention – in terms of both research and social services. Service organizations have concentrated their energies on the younger, employment-aged individual and have simultaneously ignored and underestimated the prevalence of the older population with severe vision loss (see Scott 1969). Similarly, researchers have concentrated their energies on the younger population as well – exploring obstacles to their full employment, attitudes of parents and other family members, and the like. Older persons with visual difficulties have thus become part of what Robert Scott has called the 'hidden blind.'

Blindness itself has not been a popular subject for either scholars or the general public. The topic has often been dismissed as an idiosyncratic concern, but this may well only be a way of handling our culturally inherent fear of the subject. The sighted have a documented fear of the loss of sight (Siller *et al.* 1967) which is rooted as much in culturally-imposed preconceptions of vision loss as in the actual sensory curtailment. Carlos Neu observes 'the terror of this disability is not solely the loss of an important sense; it is deeply rooted in the mythological, religious and cultural convictions' (1975: 2,161). The fears of vision loss correspond to the long tradition of portraying blindness as a sign of evil, personal transgression (especially sexual), or as punishment from the divine, perpetuated both in literature (see Monbeck 1973) and commonsensical understanding (see Scott 1969).

One consequence of scholarly and commonsense avoidance of the topic of blindness is that the literature (especially as experienced by older persons) is quite sparse. The research that does exist is often informed by the same misconceptions of blindness and vision loss found in literature and commonly held stereotypes. Furthermore, it is questionable as to just how well blindness among young persons fits the experiences of older persons with severe visual impairments. For these reasons, the study of aging and new vision-loss takes on a certain urgency.

The stories of twenty persons over age 55, each of whom lost sight in the preceding ten years, provide the data for this study (a more detailed discussion of method and methodology can be found in Appendix 1). More precisely, they all indicated that their vision loss had 'become serious enough to cause difficulties in day-to-day life' within the preceding ten years. They were all unable to read ordinary newsprint when wearing corrective lenses (a standard functional measure used to establish 'severe' vision loss). They varied in their ability to identify colors, discern light (both existence of and direction from which it comes), recognize people's facial features, and see moving objects. While they were all known to blindness agencies, they varied considerably in their exposure to services requested or received. They closely mirrored the national population of older persons who are severely impaired in terms of distribution of gender, household incomes, level of education, and cause of vision loss. Rather than unwelcome inconveniences, the differences among these people prove critical variables in understanding the natural history of vision loss. What they shared in common was both a relatively slow deterioration of vision and the corresponding threat to their sense of themselves as well as a myriad of relationships with their physical and social worlds.

The people who shared their stories of vision loss are in many ways ordinary people. They are not professional blind, *à la* Helen Keller. They have not spent their lives in schools for persons experiencing blindness nor have they been caught up in the politics of service providing/consumption that are so prevalent today. Rather, they are fathers and mothers, brothers and sisters, friends and neighbors who have experienced what many people report to be their greatest fear – the loss of sight. Their lives and their experiences will not likely receive the attention of biographers, but perhaps even more can be learned from their lives and their struggles for this very reason.

They all live in that area of the United States that we call New England. Most live in towns and small cities. In this sense, their experiences are probably somewhat different than those people living in large urban centers like New York City or the isolated countryside of Mentone, Texas. Such differences are real, and should not be minimized. They impact how persons get to the doctor, how they secure their basic needs, how easy it is to see friends and family, etc. While such issues of lifestyle and technique vary, the people who were interviewed for this study do share other things in common with people in both New York City and Mentone, Texas. They are all somewhere along a continuum of growing up and growing old. Their sense of who they are (like all people) is tied to the aging process. They understand common-sensically what has escaped many social scientists: namely, they all experience themselves as both freed and confined by their bodies, their social worlds, and their own psychological responses to both. It is this common ground that is to be explored and unpackaged here.

Ultimately, the success of any research strategy can be judged by the results that it yields. To the extent that the visually impaired older persons surveyed here are allowed to tell their own stories and the reader is able to recapture a sense of their experiences, the life histories selected for this study will prove their worth.

Who are the visually-impaired elderly?

Before unpackaging the experience of vision loss, it is necessary to take a brief detour through the language and demographics of blindness and vision loss. It would be unadvisable to begin this inquiry without some discussion of the jargon of blindness, the statistical parameters of the population, and the etiologies of age-related vision loss. To the outside and naive observer, the world of blindness will seem quite foreign. This is due, in part, to the myths and misconceptions that surround blindness and set people experiencing it apart (that they are gifted in the aesthetic arts, sensitive, have superacuity of the remaining senses, etc. – see Monbeck 1973 for a thorough review). It is, however, also due to an elaborate and technical terminology (that often eludes social scientist and person experiencing blindness alike) and a striking uncertainty as to the extent of the phenomenon among the general populace. Individuals who are experiencing the loss of vision, and their family members, are often frustrated by ophthalmologists' reluctance to explain visual disorders. This only exacerbates the sense of powerlessness and lack of control that they already feel by virtue of the vision loss itself.

Service providers are often bewildered by the differences between etiologies of vision loss among older people as well. This obscures relevant differences between consumers and may affect their ability to provide appropriate services. Their confusion regarding the extent of visual problems among older people may, likewise, impede their ability to plan programs adequately and appropriately.

Finally, as with any group, there is a language or a 'jargon' of blindness and vision loss that must be learned – if one is to become part of that group or if one simply wishes to understand it. Correspondingly, we need first to sort through the maze of terms, statistics, and clinical diagnoses that become part of the experience of blindness.

The language of blindness

As Scott (1969) has pointed out, estimating the population of people who are blind often proves a difficult task. This happens for a number of reasons, not the least of which is the often confusing language of classification by which the visual status of persons can be determined and counted. What do we mean by such expressions as 'blindness' and 'visual impairment'? The terms are often used almost interchangeably, and frequently authors do not make clear the exact nature of the visual difficulties experienced by people whose situation they seek to address.

For years, the most frequently-used standard for studying blindness was the designation 'legal' blindness. Legal blindness (in the United States) refers to a specific deterioration in eyesight as measured by clinical professionals. To qualify as legally blind one must have central visual acuity of 20/200 or less in the better eye (with best correction). This quite simply means that with best correction the person cannot see at 20 feet what a normal (20/20) person can see at 200 feet. Additionally, persons can qualify as legally blind if their field of vision is restricted to an angular distance of 20 degrees or less.

The primary alternative to using legal blindness as a standard for estimating the blind population is the National Center for Health Statistics (NCHS) measure of 'severe visual impairment.' This reflects a *subjective* reporting of *functional* vision loss – an apparent contrast with the designation of legal blindness. The NCHS measure relies on a series of interview questions asked of a national household sample that inquire into visual difficulties of the respondent. The salient responses (determining severe visual impairment) are for those persons unable to read ordinary newsprint with the aid of corrective lenses and for children under 6 years who are reported as blind in both eyes or not having useful vision in either eye.

Kirchner and Lowman (1978) observe that there are serious problems regarding the comparability of the populations. While some persons will meet both the standards of legal blindness and severe vision loss, this is often not the case. People who are legally blind are not always included in the severe visually-impaired population (not all persons who are impaired on distance vision are also impaired in near vision, and vice versa – see Kirchner and Lowman 1978: 330). Citing a 1961 report, Kirchner and Lowman (1978) report that only 38 per cent in that study qualifying for the NCHS designation as severely visually impaired would also qualify as legally blind. They further suggest that each measure may be best put to different uses. The legal-blindness designation may be better suited for generating statistics used for evaluating the need for medical services, observing epidemiological trends, or conducting research on pharmaceutical treatment, whereas the NCHS measure may be better suited to generating estimates used in policy planning and assessing the need for nonmedical services.

It is important to note that both definitions extend the population of persons experiencing severe vision-loss well beyond those who are 'totally' blind, i.e. have no remaining sight. The vast majority of legally blind and severe visually impaired people have many remaining visual skills. Many retain color and light perception, can perceive movement and/or recognize forms. Discussions of blindness must, therefore, involve populations that exceed and that are in many ways different from the narrowly-preconceived notions of blindness that most people commonsensically hold.

A final note on conceptual disparities may be in order. As if to complicate the language of blindness even further, the NCHS use of the term 'impairment' does not conform with the terminology proposed by the International Classification of Disease (Peterson, Lowman and Kirchner 1978). In these terms 'visual impairment' refers specifically to limitations in the overall functioning of the eye. It is contrasted to 'visual disability,' i.e. limitations in the ability to perform specific tasks (which would include the inability to read ordinary newsprint), 'visual disorder,' i.e. deviations from normality in the structure of the eye, and 'visual handicap,' i.e. limitations in the social functioning of the individual (a phrase that will fall into disuse given the move from 'handicap' to 'disability' as preferred language).

The demographics of age-related vision loss in the US

The ambiguities in the language of blindness are compounded by considerable statistical confusion as to the extent of vision loss. This is, of course, due partly to the lack of consensus as to which measure should be used. Depending on which classificatory scheme you use, the parameters of the population with serious visual difficulties in the United States varies.

If one uses legal blindness as the classificatory scheme by which the prevalence of blindness is estimated, the Model Reporting Area for Blindness Statistics (MRA estimates) will most likely be cited (although the MRA reporting of blindness has been discontinued and most recent estimates are from the year 1970). Established in 1962 by the National Institute of Neurological Diseases and Blindness, the MRA estimates rely on rosters of persons who are legally blind on registers maintained in a number of states. (This number has varied; in 1970 it was sixteen states. See Kirchner and Lowman 1978 for a more complete discussion of the MRA measure.)

The corresponding estimate of visual difficulties using the NCHS estimate can be found in the National Center for Health Statistics Health Interview Survey (NCHS-HIS) data. Based upon responses to an interview administered to a national random sample, NCHS-HIS data estimate the number of persons who experience severe visual impairment. These figures continue to be collected on a regular basis (every six years for the entire sample, every year for a subsample). Because the NCHS estimates continue to be compiled and because they use the growingly-popular functional measure, the NCHS-HIS figures are appearing more often in studies of blindness.

A comparison of the two data sources yields striking differences. Comparing age and gender characteristics of estimates generated by both sources, Kirchner and Lowman (1978) found, for example, that the MRA estimates greatly under-represent the elderly portion of persons with vision difficulties as well as over-represent the portion under 44 years of age. The two estimates further yield differences in terms of the gender characteristics of those with visual loss (most notably the MRA estimates indicate far fewer – 27.3 per cent as compared with 45.6 per cent – older women experiencing visual difficulties).

These disparities are consistent with Robert Scott's (1969) discovery that older persons often do not appear on state registers. Scott pointed out in his *Making of Blind Men* that there is a tendency of various counting techniques to underestimate or under-report the full extent of blindness and vision loss. Especially in the case of data using MRA estimates, a person must be formally acknowledged (registered) as blind before they will show up on the registry. This requires a recognition of the condition as well as an official clinical designation as legally blind. People who experience vision loss do have some vested interest in such a designation; tax exemptions and certain services may depend on it. For many, however, the unwillingness to acknowledge their visual difficulties or their reluctance to accept the label of 'blind' will mean that they become part of the 'hidden blind' – those who are not found on any state register. It may well be that elderly persons make up the largest single subgroup of hidden blind. This is suggested by the comparison of MRA and NCHS-HIS estimates. It can probably be explained by the relatively few benefits accorded older persons who are blind (hence reducing the incentive to be registered) as well as a stronger sense of revulsion at the official designation. The NCHS-HIS estimates are not as susceptible to this difficulty, but are vulnerable precisely because they do reflect subjective evaluations of an individual's visual condition. For some purposes, this too limits their usefulness. In any case, this obviously makes the demographics of blindness and vision loss even more problematic. One can, however, safely assume that the full extent of visual difficulties probably exceeds any statistical estimates (Kirchner and Peterson 1979: 72 arrive at a similar conclusion). With all this in mind, however, it is likely that the NCHS-HIS estimates are considerably better (however flawed they may be because of the problems with self-reporting) in discussing the elderly who experience visual losses.

The demographics of the elderly population in the US necessarily speak to the demographics of the phenomenon of age-related vision problems. According to estimates based on the NCHS-HIS data from 1977, 44.5 per 1,000 persons over age 65 experience severe visual impairment (Kirchner and Peterson 1979). Applying this to the 25 million persons who were over age 65 in 1980, we can translate this into more than 1 million persons. Changing the statistical focus, older persons who are blind or who experience severe vision loss are also of particular interest because they constitute most of the total population so designated. Of all those persons who are registered as legally blind in the US, those over 65 represent 46.2 per cent (Kirchner and Lowman 1978). If one uses the figures on severe vision loss reported by NCHS, the figures are even more striking; 67.7 per cent of all those who report severe vision loss are over age 65 (Kirchner and Lowman 1978).

Looking to the future, as the population of persons over age 65 continues to swell, so too will the numbers of older persons experiencing severe visual impairment. By the year 2000 it is estimated that the number of persons over 65 who are severely visually impaired will be 1,756,000 (this compares to MRA estimates of the legally-blind elderly in the year 2000 of just 272,000 persons, see Kirchner and Lowman 1978). Notably, the greatest changes will come in the age 85-and-over segment of the elderly, which will increase by 84 per cent over the 1977 population (and whose prevalence rate of visual impairment is 181.5 per 1,000 persons, as compared with a rate of 22 per 1,000 persons among those 65–74).

The eyes and the aging process

While one will be constantly frustrated in a search for the best measure of the prevalence of visual difficulties among the elderly, the issue of physiological etiology can be more readily settled. The terminology is equally technical, however, and serves as a constant frustration to persons trying to find out information about the troubles they or another family member are having with their eyes.

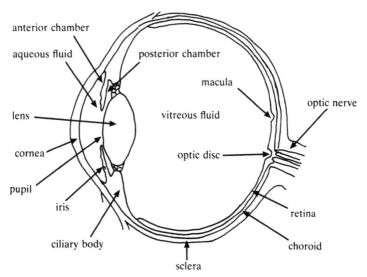

anterior chamber

aqueous fluid

posterior chamber

macula

optic nerve

lens

vitreous fluid

cornea

optic disc

pupil

iris

retina

ciliary body

choroid

sclera

Figure 1.1 Cutaway view of the normal eye

The eye is, of course, a 'dual organ,' in that two normally functioning eyes are required for normal vision (Eden 1978). It is composed of numerous and highly specialized cells, as well as its own muscle, fibrous connective, and nervous systems. Figure 1.1 offers a cutaway view of the eye's major components. As can be seen, the eye is elliptical in shape and has three distinct concentric tissue layers – the sclera, uveal tract, and retina.

The first and outermost layer, composed of the sclera and cornea, is largely protective in nature. The **cornea** is a transparent layer which lies in front of the pupil and iris (which will be discussed more fully in a moment). The **sclera** is the so-called 'white of the eye' which covers the remaining five-sixths of the eye's surface.

The second layer, lying just beneath the outer protective layer, is the **uveal tract** and its main purposes are circulatory and muscular. The second layer's chief components are the iris, the ciliary body, and the choroid. The **iris** is the round, colored part of the eye surrounding the **pupil** (which is simply a hole through which light enters the inner eye). The iris facilitates the passing of light into the eye by constricting in bright light to make the pupil smaller and dilating in dimmer light to make the pupil larger. The **ciliary body** lies next to the iris and contracts or relaxes to alter the shape of the eye's lens. It is, therefore, the mechanism which allows the eye to focus on objects of varying distances from the observer. The ciliary body is the focusing muscle of the eye. The ciliary body also secretes the **aqueous fluid** (or aqueous humor – the watery fluid filling the anterior and posterior chambers of the eye – which nourishes and lubricates the lens and cornea). Next to the ciliary body in this second layer of the eye is the **choroid**. It is the main circulatory mechanism of the eye. Small arteries carry blood to portions of the eye requiring it for their metabolism, and veins return with carbon dioxide waste.

The third and final concentric layer of the eye is the **retina**. It is an extremely thin sheet of nerve tissue which receives visual images (including size, shape, dimension, position in space, relative distance, and color) and transmits them, via the optic nerve, to the visual center of the brain. The retina has several major subcomponents as well. The most notable of these is the **macula**. The macula is responsible for a person's sharp central vision (i.e. permits normal 20/20 visual acuity) while the rest of the retina's surface is responsible for receiving peripheral visual images. While most of the retina's surface is serviced by blood vessels, the central portion of the macular region (or fovea) is not. It is, by contrast, entirely free of blood vessels. This characteristic of the macula insures that it is unobstructed by blood vessels but also makes it more vulnerable to damage than the rest of the retina (this, as will be seen, is especially pertinent to many age-related eye disorders). The retina also has specialized cells which enable the eye to adapt to light changes and color distinctions. Cells called **rods** are sensitive to low intensities of light while **cones** are those cells sensitive to higher intensities of light (cones are also responsible for color distinction).

Within these three concentric layers of the eye are the **optical media**. The optical media are the clear structures lying between the cornea (at the front of the eye) and the retina (upon which visual images are received at the back of the eye). The cornea, at the frontmost part of the optical media, is unobstructed (like the macula) by blood vessels. It is covered with tears on its outside surface and the aqueous fluid (secreted by the ciliary body as mentioned earlier) on its inside surface. These two fluids are constantly secreted and then drained away from the eye (again, in the drainage of the aqueous fluid, this is particularly relevant to age-related visual disorders). The aqueous fluid, as described earlier, lies between the cornea and the next component of the optical media, the **lens**. The normal lens is perfectly transparent and is flexible, which allows a person to focus on objects at both a distance and near at hand. Like the cornea, there is no vascular system in the lens and it too receives its nourishment from the aqueous fluid. The center of the eye is filled with the last major component of the optical media, the **vitreous fluid**. Unlike the aqueous fluid, the vitreous fluid is neither manufactured nor circulated but is rather a stable gel-like mass. Its major function is to retain the shape and resilience of the eye while allowing light to pass to the retinal surface.

These concentric layers, circulatory, macular, and nervous systems, and internal structures make up the major components of the normal eye. As will be seen, many of these components are susceptible to changes prompted by aging of the human organism. It is these changes which, in the more severe instances, can lead to a drastic curtailment of the individual's visual capacity.

Some of the common age-related changes in the eye are as follows. The cornea begins to flatten with age, which leads to the commonly-experienced astigmatism of the eyes (an optical error resulting in two instead of one point of focus, which manifests itself in a blurring of vision – see Kasper 1983: 479). The sclera becomes less elastic and takes on a more yellow coloration due to fatty depositions (Kasper 1983: 479). The drainage system (trabecular meshwork), by which the aqueous fluid is allowed to leave the eye, thickens and a sclerosis of the tissue occurs such that the free circulation of the aqueous fluid is hampered (in more severe instances, as will be discussed, this can contribute to glaucoma – see Halasa 1972). Connective tissue in the uveal tract thickens and becomes more diffuse. The iris, in particular, attains a rigid character resulting in a smaller pupil which, in part, explains the need often experienced by older persons for more light to read (see Coni *et al.* 1977: 279). The lens of the eye often loses its ability to increase in thickness and curvature, resulting in presbyopia which inhibits the eye's capacity to focus on near objects (hence the common need for bifocals in persons over 40 – see Coni *et al.* 1977; Kasper 1983). In addition to these changes in the uveal tract, the retina also commonly goes through a series of age-related changes. Most commonly, these changes affect the retinal circulation. Arterioles and veins, for example, often become narrowed (Kasper 1983: 480). Frequently 'floaters' begin to appear as well in the vitreous fluid, giving the appearance of 'dots,' 'lines,' or 'cobwebs' to the older person. Changes in the external portion of the eye can also compound age-related changes in the internal eye. The eyelid can wrinkle and suffer decreases in muscle tone, with the effect that the eyelash interferes with the cornea. Tear secretion can also decrease with age, hence causing discomfort and severe inflammation (Kasper 1983: 481).

As has been suggested, these age-related changes in the eye do not lead to serious vision loss in most people. There is some reason to believe that more people would experience serious vision loss if it were not for mortality. J.S. Friedenwald (1952), for instance, has gone so far as to suggest that blindness would be universal if human survival were extended to 130 years. At present, of course, this is not the case. Yet for some people these changes of the eye lead to severe impairments in their visual capacity.

One of the most common causes of severe visual disorder in aging individuals is the **cataract**. It can be defined as any opacification or loss of transparency in the lens of the eye (Eden 1978: 186). Kasper suggests that over 95 per cent of all persons over age 65 have cataracts to some degree (1983: 481). For most people, however, these cataracts never become advanced enough to cause severe visual loss in their lifetime. Although it is so common, the mechanism of the formation of cataracts is not known (Kasper 1983: 481).

Quite simply, the lens of the normal eye (as with the other optical media) is clear and allows light to pass through on its way to the retina. Thus, any imperfection of the lens can affect vision. The size and density of opacifications vary greatly and so too does the effect on vision. In some instances the filters of the lens become compressed toward its center, resulting in nuclear sclerosis and the beginning of a senile cataract (Kornzweig 1979: 379). In other instances cataract formation is characterized by groups or opaque spokes of lens fibers which, for one reason or another, lose their transparency (Kornzweig 1979: 379). The net result of cataracts of all varieties is a blurring of vision. Yet the cataract can cause this blurring of vision to varying degrees. If they are minimal, the person may be able to look past them with near normal vision. In the case of more substantial cataract formations persons may feel like they are looking through 'smoked' or 'steamed' glass. In still more advanced or substantial cataract formations, it may become impossible to see anything.

The only known successful treatment for the cataract is the surgical removal of the cataract lens. Performed by a properly-trained surgeon, this procedure is estimated to be close to 95 to 98 per cent successful (Kornzweig 1979: 370). Yet a large portion of those people suffering from cataract formations either postpone or avoid indefinitely this surgery, and live instead with the visual consequences.

A second major cause of severe visual disorder is **glaucoma**. Glaucoma takes several forms, but is typically characterized by an elevation of intraocular pressure (Kasper 1983: 482). This change in intraocular pressure is almost always related to changes in or around the anterior chamber angle of the eye which controls the normal outflow of the aqueous fluid. It will be recalled that the aqueous fluid is secreted by the ciliary body and fills both the anterior and posterior chambers of the eye. It is drained from the eye by filtering through the trabecular meshwork (at the angle or end point of the anterior chamber – see Figure 1.1) into what is called Schlemm's canal which, in turn, allows the aqueous fluid to enter the blood system. For the eye to maintain a steady level of intraocular pressure, the outflow rate of the aqueous fluid must be equal to its rate of inflow (Halasa 1972: 17). Glaucoma develops because the rate of absorption of the aqueous fluid into the bloodstream is reduced abnormally; hence, intraocular pressure increases. Specifically, Halasa estimates that 99 per cent of all glaucoma results from obstructions in the trabecular meshwork (1972: 65). This obstruction is usually caused by extraordinary thickening of the trabecular fibers.

The elevation in intraocular pressure affects the eye in several ways. The increasing pressure makes the eye harder and causes stress in all its parts. In particular, however, it is most threatening to the delicate nerve fibers of the optic nerve (which transmits sensory data from the retina to the brain). If the increased pressure caused by glaucoma remains unchecked, it kills the nerve fibers in the optic nerve. Those on the outer edge of the optic disc are the first to die. Progressively, cells further toward the center are killed as well. Thus, with glaucoma, the peripheral visual field continually narrows. Persons suffering from glaucoma therefore often complain of and experience tunnel vision and are unable to see anything off to the sides of their center vision. If glaucoma is allowed to run its course, eventually even this center vision will be lost as well. Ironically, it is possible for persons with some remaining center vision to have 20/20 vision acuity when looking at something straight ahead of them.

It is estimated that from 2 per cent (Veirs 1970: 26) to 4 per cent (Eden 1978: 132) of people over age 40 have chronic simple glaucoma. Kornzweig (1979) estimates that 5 per cent of people over age 65 have glaucoma. It cannot be prevented or cured, but can usually be effectively controlled (Eden 1978: 137). Damage caused by glaucoma cannot be repaired, so early diagnosis is considered essential. Eyedrops which either enlarge the drainage angle or inhibit secretion of aqueous fluid are the most common treatment for glaucoma.

Many instances of age-related severe visual-impairments are caused by changes in the retina. Quite frequently, these changes affect the macular portion of the retina (again, that portion responsible for clear center vision) through sclerosis of the choroidal arteries (in part responsible for the nourishment of the macula), severe hypertension, diabetes, nervous system conditions such as multiple sclerosis, and vascular thrombosis, as well as many other unknown causes (Kornzweig 1979: 375). Such factors often lead to a degeneration of the macula and a loss in central vision. Quite appropriately, these are referred to as instances of **macular degeneration**.

Curiously, the problems for the person with macular degeneration can be just the reverse of the person suffering from glaucoma. With glaucoma, as noted above, the person may retain normal central vision and lose peripheral vision. Persons experiencing macular degeneration will lose their central vision but their peripheral vision can often be unaffected. The result is that, with macular degeneration, such tasks as distinguishing the features of other people's faces, reading, and doing detailed work become extremely difficult, if not impossible (Kornzweig 1979: 375).

Persons with macular degeneration are often targeted for the use of low-vision aids. Such items as magnifying glasses for close work, telescopic lenses to improve distance vision, and closed-circuit televisions which dramatically increase the size of the printed word are often effective ways of aiding the person with macular degeneration. Treatment for the condition itself, however, has been largely ineffective (Kornzweig 1979; Kasper 1983).

One specific cause of retinal disorders worthy of individual mention is **diabetic retinopathy**. Persons who have had diabetes for more than ten years are particularly prone to have haemorrhages in the retina which often affect the macula (Kornzweig 1979: 376). Indeed, the loss of sight associated with diabetes is so common that it is 'virtually diagnostic of the disease' (Kasper 1983: 485). It is estimated that diabetes affects about 20 per cent of the population over age 65 in western societies, so the worthiness of singling out diabetic retinopathy should be readily apparent (Williams 1978: 327). Specifically, diabetes affects the retina by causing damage to its blood vessels. Some vessels become plugged, others leak fluid, while still others grow abnormally along the inner surface of the retina. Often the damage to the retina's vessels may lead to what is called a vitreous haemorrhage, in which fluid leaks into the vitreous itself, thus interfering with the passage of the light to the retinal surface.

One of the most severe ways that diabetic retinopathy affects vision is by producing a **retinal detachment**. On occasion, the newly-formed blood vessels on the retinal surface can lead to an actual shrinkage of the vitreous and/or scar tissue on the retina. In such instances the retina is pulled away from the choroid. This can even cause the retina to tear (Eden 1978: 111).

A retinal detachment can also be caused by cataract surgery. It is estimated that such detachment occurs in about 2 per cent of cases (Kasper 1983: 485). Regardless of the cause, the symptoms of retinal detachment are the experience of flashes of light, the distortion of images and an often rapid loss of sight. If not treated quickly, the retinal detachment almost always gets worse; the detached area gets larger and/or the retina may tear away from the choroid in several places. Treatment is always surgical and is usually accomplished either by cauterizing or freezing the tear to reattach the retina to the choroid.

A wide variety of **vascular occlusions** can also lead to vision loss. Vascular disease of both extracranial and intracranial blood vessels (both prone to occur in aged persons) can lead to minor or even serious eye disorders. Most serious are occlusions to the central retinal artery. When retinal circulation is blocked, the cells of the retina begin to die which, in turn, reduces its capacity to receive and send visual images to the brain. The cells which are affected may either be on the periphery of the retina or near the macula and, correspondingly, affect either peripheral or center vision, or both.

One last cause of vision loss which needs to be mentioned is **retinitis pigmentosa**. Unlike the other causes of new vision loss treated above, retinitis pigmentosa is not actually prompted by the biological changes in the organism accompanying the process of aging. Rather, it is a hereditary disease of the eyes. Retinitis pigmentosa begins in young adulthood but only progressively reaches levels of severe vision loss when people reach middle or advanced age (which justifies its inclusion in this section – see J. Parsons 1970: 327ff.). The disease is first evident in people's late teens with the onset of night blindness. Progressively, the visual field begins to constrict and, like glaucoma, peripheral vision is lost first (Parsons 1970: 328). Finally, people usually lose center vision as well by the time they are around age 60.

Retinitis pigmentosa affects primarily the rods and the cones (particularly the former – see J. Parsons 1970: 328). It will be recalled that the rods are those cells in the retina which are sensitive to low light-intensities, which explains the prevalence of night blindness in retinitis pigmentosa's early stages. Again, the macular region is not usually affected until the late stages of the disease. With retinitis pigmentosa, the retinal arterioles become attenuated, the optic disc typically atrophies, and eventually posterior cataracts form and choroidal sclerosis occurs (Scheie and Albert 1969: 131). Retinal cells are replaced by pigmented tissue which, upon examination, takes on the appearance of a 'crow having walked across the retina' (Chalkley 1974: 58). Glaucoma itself is a frequent complication of the disease (Chalkley 1974: 59). Regrettably, there is no known way to alter the course of retinitis pigmentosa (Weinstein 1977: 3).

Beyond the physiology of vision loss

In brief, then, these are the major categories of age-related vision loss. They have been outlined in some detail so as to stress that there are, indeed, physiological changes that occur in the aging eye itself. While the ensuing analysis will focus upon the subjective accounts of people who are visually impaired, this is not to suggest that new vision loss is an ethereal product. Vision loss is, on the contrary, prompted by one of several concrete biological processes. Yet these processes, labels, and numbers are given human meaning only when understood as mediated by the individual's own experiences and interpretations of vision loss. These experiences and interpretations must be, in turn, understood in relation to the social context in which the individual is located. In fact, when proportioned out, the physiological roots of vision loss may be the least salient to understanding the experience. The individual's fears, personally- and socially-imposed limitations, and the re-actions of other people overwhelm and often exaggerate the physiological loss itself.

Correspondingly, the experience of vision loss dictates a certain order to the book. Chapter 2 takes up people's response to the physiological changes that are imposed by the loss of sight. It traces people's experience of its progression – their awareness of, reactions to, and explanations of vision loss. Chapter 2 also explores people's accounts of the limitations to activity that are imposed, preconceptions of blindness and those who experience it, and the ways in which they have to reorganize their lives, sense of self, and basic categories of experience such as time and space.

Chapter 3 examines the visually-impaired person in relation to the social world – of family, friends, service providers, other people who are visually impaired – that surrounds them. It traces the impact of vision loss on the interactive process. It also outlines the reactions of others to the loss of sight – from the protective response of family members to the avoidance reaction of old friends. Chapter 3 reveals changes in people's social networks that are prompted by vision loss. It also takes account of socially-imposed limitations to activity as well as the critical advisory roles that other people play in people's adjustment.

Chapter 4 then explores the various means by which people attempt to make sense of their losses (the physical loss itself, as well as lost plans, lost friends, and, in some cases, lost self). How can the loss be contextualized? How do people explain away an event that 'never could happen to them'? These and other questions that bear upon the classic Weberian issue of legitimation are reviewed in Chapter 4.

The final chapter, Chapter 5, places the experience of vision loss within the larger context of aging and lifelong physiological, social, and psychological change. It unfolds, if you will, the larger implications of age-related vision loss for our understanding of human aging (conceived of as a process that extends throughout the life course and that is not restricted to late life alone).

Chapter two

Contending with the advent of vision loss

A person's experiences of the world and self are bound up with her/his experience of her/his body. To borrow from the phenomenological philosophers, all of human experience is 'embodied' experience. At the risk of stating the obvious, the body necessarily accompanies a person through all aspects of her/his involvement in the world. It anchors the individual in a world of things and other people. The body enables the person to grasp a fork to eat her/his food, to move from one side of the street to the other, and it likewise allows interaction with other people. While this may seem commonsensically apparent, it is a fundamental beginning point for understanding human experience that has escaped the attention of many social scientists.

A person's ties to her/his body are perhaps made most clear when something about the body goes awry. A simple headache reminds people that even the most modest bodily disturbance can affect the way that they see the world, their willingness to take on new projects, or their ability to deal with stressful situations. So fundamental is bodily experience to human beings that, to a considerable degree, people's sense of who they are is tied to their bodies. As R.D. Laing (1960: 66) puts it, 'in ordinary circumstances, to the extent that one feels one's body to be alive, real and substantial, one feels oneself alive, real and substantial.'

People are, in other words, aware that the body both enables and limits their intentions. They are aware of using their bodies as tools to accomplish their goals and they are equally aware of bodily limitations. Even the tallest person will at one time or another come across something that is out of reach. The experience of something out of reach simultaneously tells the person that the body enables (it is the vehicle by which one can grasp things in the first place) and limits (body is too short to accomplish her/his intention – that is, her/his intentions exceed the body). It is even quite possible that a person can feel 'trapped' inside a body which is experienced as an inadequate reflection of the consciousness within it. This has been suggested of dwarfs (Truzzi 1968), the visibly disabled (Davis 1964), the facially disfigured (Bernstein 1975), and of individuals experiencing 'anosognosia' (the denial of illness, Shontz 1975).

None of this is intended to suggest that bodily experience explains the whole of what it means to be human. Peter Berger and Thomas Luckmann (1966: 50) describe people's relationship to their bodies as 'eccentric.' By this they mean that while every movement is tied to a body – hence consciousness and body are coextensive – people are not identical with their bodies. While they realize that their bodies are indispensable, they also realize that their bodies do not express the whole of who they are. In fact, they often feel that they have their bodies 'at their disposal.' This is to say that they view their bodies as subject to manipulation by some other aspect of self. Most people are aware then – whether they view their bodies as enabling or limiting – of both being and having a body.

All of this is critical to understanding both the aging experience generally, and vision loss more specifically. While a person is not identical with her/his body, the changes that occur to her/his body clearly affect the nature of experience. Since the body both enables and limits, changes in the body over the course of a lifetime can alter what is within and out of reach (literally and figuratively). Aging involves, by definition, a variety of physiological changes, whether one examines infancy, adolescence, or old age. Just as the infant must learn to develop physiological equilibrium, eye–hand coordination, and the like, the adolescent must come to terms with the dramatic physical changes of puberty, and the older person must adjust to a number of physiological changes that are markers of late life. Despite the reluctance of social scientists to recognize its importance, bodily experience is a critical beginning point in understanding human aging – not that it exhausts the phenomenon by any means, but rather because all of human aging refers to bodily experience.

Changes in visual acuity are precisely what define the population of persons who are visually impaired – hence the need in the preceding chapter to spend time on the various etiologies of vision loss. This is not to say that the physiological changes of age-related vision loss are the major features of the experience. The various etiologies of vision loss accompanying the aging process do not occur within an experiential vacuum. On the contrary, the physiological changes which occur in the deterioration of the eye carry with them a host of experiences for people which force them to rethink their lives, their future, their past, their bodies, and even how they see themselves. All of these experiences – many of which center on relations with other people – ultimately outweigh the physical loss itself. To set the stage for the discussion of those experiences, it is both necessary and appropriate to begin by reviewing the initial progression of vision loss, the initial changes in bodily experience.

The progression of vision loss

People often seem surprised to learn that the loss of sight isn't usually sudden or violent. This surprise is likely due, in part, to most people's fear, as well as their misunderstandings, of blindness. Most commonly, the first signs of new vision loss occur while the individual is carrying on routine day-to-day activities. There is seldom a single dramatic point at which the person no longer sees. This certainly can happen – as is the case in some trauma-related blindness – but it is unusual. Rather, the first signs of vision loss are characteristically slow in developing and often dismissed as the product of 'tired eyes' or a day 'overdone,' until the impairment can no longer be denied. A person experiencing macular degeneration describes her first awareness of her impending vision loss:

A year ago last January, when we were in Arizona visiting my sister-in-law, I noticed that she had a big clock on the wall and things seemed a little hazy to me. So, you know how you cover one eye and look? Well, I covered the left eye and I could see fine, but when I covered the right eye I couldn't see out of the left eye. The face of the clock – it was a big clock – the face of it was all black. I thought for a while that maybe I was tired or something like that. But it didn't go away. So after a couple of weeks, I came home and I saw Dr Arnold and he said that I had ruptured a vessel. He said that it might seal over and heal itself some but if it didn't I should seek further advice on it. Well, my sight came back and it seemed to improve some. If I was tired, I'd have trouble and I couldn't see quite as much. But, ah, during the summer, I could read different things we had around so I figured that it was to a point, you know, where that was it.

This person's hope that her vision difficulties had stabilized soon proved to be unfounded. Like so many others, she would continue to have some days when her eyesight would appear to improve but more often it would be all too apparent that it was steadily getting worse. For most people the loss will be gradual and for most it will

23

never be complete – that is, they will always have some remaining sight.

Because the loss of sight accompanying the aging process is usually gradual rather than sudden, it does not neatly fit into the traditional social-psychological concern with 'crisis situations' which has attracted the attention of students of identity. Fred Davis (1963), for example, defines a crisis situation as 'a relatively sudden and unanticipated disruption, of extensive and protracted significance, in the everyday activities, understandings and expectations of a social unit' (1963: 17). Certainly the loss of sight meets most of Davis' criteria, i.e. vision loss is usually unanticipated, it is definitely of extensive and protracted significance, and, as will be shown, it certainly disrupts the everyday activities, understandings, and expectations of both people experiencing vision loss and those around them. It is, however, often drawn out over a number of years. Nevertheless, new vision loss demands the reappraisal of one's life course (past, present, future) which Davis and others (see Anselm Strauss' discussion of turning points, 1969: 100ff.) have argued to be the essential characteristic of the crisis situation. Thus, the actual process by which sight is lost follows a gradual path of decline, but this does not lessen the import of these reappraisals, nor does it soften the impact of this sensory loss upon the person's daily life.

Quite often, having no reason to suspect that they are suffering from serious eye disorders, people look for typical age-related disorders to explain away the initial signs of vision loss. They frequently turn to the readily-acceptable explanation that their eye glasses need changing (a routine exercise to many aging persons). As if to cling to the 'normal' decline of her cohort, another person reported that she hoped that high blood pressure was causing her eye problems.

> I knew that something was wrong because I would miss a step or turn around and run into things. See, I lost the sight on the sides first, which is typical. And then I thought at first it was, you know, a blood pressure problem. . . . I would sort of lose my balance a little bit, or turn sideways quick and lost it. Sometimes I wouldn't see a step or something like that. This was the first of it. But I wasn't too alarmed because, like I said, I thought it was blood pressure. . . . So I went and had all these blood tests taken and everything and found that I did have fat in my blood, you know? Cholesterol. I had to take some medicine and my blood was fine after some more tests. But I said 'But my eyes are no better. In fact, I think they're worse.'

'Cholesterol,' 'high blood pressure,' 'fatigue' – these and other colloquial diagnoses allow vision difficulties to be placed within the realm of routine problems. There is something more – or perhaps less – than 'denial' involved in this search for a diagnosis that a person considers typical of their age group. For most people, there is really no reason to suspect that their new-found troubles with seeing owe anything to a chronic visual problem. Hence the shock with which they receive the official medical diagnosis becomes all the more understandable. In the case of the individual above, once referred to an eye specialist, it became quite clear that she was experiencing the early warning signs of retinitis pigmentosa. While retinitis pigmentosa is a hereditary disease, it often skips generations, and sometimes, as in the case of this individual, persons can be quite unaware of the vision loss which awaits them. This failure to anticipate visual decline is not only common to people with retinitis pigmentosa but is characteristic of those experiencing other forms of vision loss as well. Only when their eyes fail to focus, or they misjudge distances, or fail to see objects in their near environment, do people suspect that something is wrong with their eyes. Furthermore, in most cases, the gravity of their visual difficulties only becomes clear when confirmed by a battery of tests which are common to early vision loss.

> I went to the specialist and of course he could tell right off that something was drastically wrong with my retina. Because he didn't have the necessary machines, I had to go to Boston. It was a pretty drastic experience, to say the least, you know? To go down there – and they took all kinds of pictures of the eye and enlarged them. First they inject this dye into your system, in your blood system and so forth and that's when they told me it was retinitis pigmentosa. And then, from then on, it seemed to go faster. If someone accidentally left the cupboard door open, I would run into it. I would turn around quickly and run into the refrigerator or run into my husband – they're both big. Well, you know my husband, he said 'Well something's drastically wrong when you can't see me.' It actually went gradually. I could see the difference from one year to the next, you know, on the amount that I could see.

Eventually, then, the hope that a person's visual problems are rooted in some normal abnormality, a characteristic decline of her/ his age cohort, gives way to the recognition that she/he is now beginning the life of a person with a visual impairment.

Unlike persons with retinitis pigmentosa, many people who become adventitiously visually impaired have some medical or surgical recourse by which their disorder can be approached. Cataracts can be surgically removed, the intraocular pressure of glaucoma can often be controlled and, in some cases, even the rather drastic detachment of the retina can be at least partially corrected. Waiting and hoping, therefore, become major pre-occupations.

Many people find themselves 'awaiting surgery,' 'waiting for cataracts to "ripen"' (a strange and misleading description of cataracts that is often used to explain a decision to put off surgery), 'hoping a new medication will be more effective.' Like all waiting, these situations remind the person of her/his lack of power in the situation. As Schwartz (1975, 1978) reports, it is the general rule that people without power await the powerful. Poor blacks have to wait longer than affluent whites, patients wait on doctors, and the employee waits on the employer. This fundamental message regarding waiting and power/powerlessness is not lost on the person experiencing vision loss. They will not only have to wait on potential remedies, but they will also have to wait in the office of their ophthalmologist for service providers to pay them a visit, and for family members or friends to understand that vision loss hasn't really changed them as a person.

Be this as it may, for many people the progression of vision loss is inseparable from the corrective procedures which simultaneously provide so much hope, consume so much time, and, in some cases, supply so much pain. With apparent resignation, one man recalled the failed attempts to reattach his retina.

When it started it left a spot in the eye and see with the degeneration I didn't have no more sight in the center of the eye, you know? If I would look at anything, right at it, like if I'd look at a traffic light, I wouldn't see it. I would have to turn my head a little. See my peripheral vision was a lot better than my central vision. Then the real big thing came in November of 1970 when I had a total detachment in my right eye. It took about a week. It started in the corner but see my eye is elongated like an egg, it is not round, you know? So that kind of stretched everything, so when the little corner of the retina started to detach, it took about a week until the thing was gone. I saw the doctor then and he started to make arrangements for me in Boston to have an operation. It took about a week and then they took a chance to operate. They told me before the operation that the chance was very small but I had lost the sight in the eye so I didn't have nothing to lose. The doctor said 'we can try to put it back.' See, they had to go inside the eye to push the retina back. Like I say, my eye was stretched so they had to take – it was a fine needle – a needle with a little balloon at the end and they blew that up to put the retina back. To try and seal it back there, you know? They burned it with a laser beam to make a scar. But the operation was not successful on account of hemorrhaging. Maybe the operation was all right but the eye hemorrhaged and there was nothing they could do. After that they tried to pack the eye to remove some of the blood but it started hemorrhaging again so we had to give it up.

For those whose vision loss has progressed to some considerable degree and for whom there are no medical or surgical remedies (or those which have been tried and proved unsuccessful), the recollection of the onset of their vision loss is beset most frequently with such resignation. Sometimes, however, resignation gives way to bitterness and discouragement, as is apparent in the case of an individual with glaucoma who recalls his treatment.

I should say about six or seven years ago I could see something was wrong. I made an appointment with a doctor who has a really good reckoning in this part of the country. Well, he treated me, oh, half a dozen times. He done me a lot of good at the start. He cleared me up in good vision. Then things started to go caput and it's been getting worse ever since. Two years ago, last September, then, I was operated on. Well to me it looks as if he dug in there and shook things around. All around. And he left dirt in there. He didn't take that stuff off. It looks as if there was dirt all over my eye, in other words. That's what it looks like to me. But apparently there is nothing they can do about it. After they operated on me in September, he had a patch over this eye for about three weeks. Then he gave me a prescription for three different pairs of glasses. The last one was eighty-five dollars. The others were fifty dollars or something like that. I forget now. Well, anyway, none of those glasses is any good. That is, it didn't help me anyway. So that's why I got so god damned discouraged.

For those persons for whom surgical or medical remedies still hold out some hope, the recollection of the past progression of vision loss is often tempered by hope for future improvements.

In July I went to see Dr Morton because I had seen floaters. I guess that's what they call them – floaters. And he said there was nothing that he could do about it. But when I went again in November, he discovered that I had a cataract in this eye. We had planned to have it removed last month but I came down with a bleeding ulcer in my stomach. So right now I'm supposed to go back. I'm supposed to go in January if everything goes all right and have this cataract removed. I asked him if I would see again. He said 'Yes,' he said that 'I can promise that you will see about as good as you did in the spring.' In the spring, I could read a letter. Now I can't even see the top line of anything. And I can't see your face. You know how close you are? [about four feet] I don't even know what you have for a face at all. I can't recognize my own children. Oh, how I hope to be well enough to go in January to have this cataract removed. He promised me that I would see a little bit better.

This person, like all others, recounted the numerous difficulties associated with her ongoing visual decline yet she (unlike those for whom surgical and medical remedies held little if any promise) hastily added the emphatic hope that her vision would improve.

Quite often one cause of vision impairment may be controlled, only to discover that another age-related disorder remains unchecked. Therefore, in discussing the progression of vision loss, people often have to account for more than one visual problem. For example, one person discovered that her difficulties were due to both glaucoma and macular degeneration. The glaucoma disrupted her peripheral vision while the macular degeneration impacted upon her center vision. While the former was eventually brought under control, the latter steadily affects her sight.

I always had good eyes until about six years ago. Six or seven years ago. I had good eyesight before that. Well, I had my eyes checked for glaucoma. I didn't even know I had it. They started putting in drops and trying to control, you know, both eyes. I had it really in my right eye but he [the doctor] told me that usually when you have it in one eye you have it in the other. Well, he said that if I should go up in the left eye then it won't damage that eye because I'm using these drops. They work good for me so the pressure is good in both eyes now.

But my eyesight kept getting worse and then they found out that I was getting this blind spot in the center of my eye. I got it in my left, now I got it in both. I think that is worse than the glaucoma. The pressure, I can control it good but this other thing, I can't do anything about it, you know? If I look straight ahead at anything I am blind, you know? But then, whatever I want to see, I just move my sight to the side of it and then I see. Of course, it's not plain. I can't see it too well but that is the only way that I can see at all. It is too bad that I had to come down with this other thing. It is really a worse bother. They tell

me that I won't go totally blind but with the two problems, you
know, it worries me.

Thus vision loss is not clearly the result of one cause or another but
rather may be due to a series of physiological changes occurring
simultaneously in the aging eye. Furthermore, people often find
their loss of vision accompanied by other changes in the body as a
whole. Often this leaves people confused about the causes of their
new-found difficulties.

In their initial efforts to make sense of the vision loss, people
usually attempt to trace their vision difficulties to specific
behaviors, situations, or events. A woman, medically diagnosed as
having macular degeneration, for example, reported that her
visual difficulties were due to her overexposure to smoke which
resulted from an instance when she failed to open the chimney flue
before starting a fire. Another person, also diagnosed as having
macular degeneration, reported that his eye difficulties were due
to 'close work' he had had to do while working in a factory which
'strained' his eyes. Fitzgerald (1971) found that this is common
among recently-blind adults and discovered that over half of the
people he studied had such commonsensical understandings of
their vision loss.

These attempts to explain the origins of vision loss are part of
the concerted effort that all people make to 'make sense' of the
world around them. People presume that their lives are more than
random events – that there is a certain causal order that, if
discovered, makes sense of it all. Typical of most 'good fortune'
and 'misfortune,' people find it difficult to believe that things
simply happen or that people profit or suffer without reason (see
Ainlay and Crosby 1986). Explanations extend from these sort of
commonsensical accounts to lay theories of divine justice (this will
be discussed in greater detail). For the person who loses her/his
sight, it can no more be considered a random occurrence than the
death of a child or a job promotion. Often the process of
discovering the source of vision loss proves evasive, but whether
found or in search of, all people look for the order that causal
explanations provide.

An additional note on the progression of vision loss is essential.
The markedly gradual and often confusing loss of sight leaves most
people with some remaining vision. Indeed, all but a tiny fraction
of people with blindness have some remaining vision. Most retain
at least some remaining light perception or can still distinguish
forms and movement (although with pronounced difficulty). This
remaining sight, however slight it might be, often proves very

important to people's ability to orient themselves spatially. The light from windows, for example, can be used to place oneself in a room. Thus, for most older people experiencing new vision loss, the world is one of reduced (rather than totally eliminated) visual cues. This is important to bear in mind as one discusses their engagement of the world around them.

The curtailment of activities

There is little doubt that people with sight impose their misconceptions regarding its loss upon those who actually experience it. In large part, these misconceptions may flow from the fears sighted people have about blindness. Michael Monbeck (1973) has discussed two different sorts of misconceptions that characterize attitudes toward blindness. On the one hand, there are those that are 'primary' – that is, misconceptions that emphasize various kinds and degrees of loss. On the other, there are those that are 'secondary' – that is, misconceptions that emphasize the effects of these losses on the individual. An example of primary attitudinal misconceptions would be that blindness means total darkness. Examples of secondary misconceptions would be that blindness leads a person to become more inner-directed or to have greater appreciation of music and other aesthetic activities. Monbeck insists that both primary and secondary attitudinal misconceptions have quite negative implications for the experience of blindness. Ralph Riffenburgh (1967: 127) has noted that misunderstandings even inform the attitudes and emotional response of service workers for the blind and, hence, block their ability to evaluate people's situation realistically. (Monbeck suggests it is particularly ironic that so many service agencies have chosen the name 'Lighthouse' – a fairly obvious play on the primary misconception of blindness as darkness.) These images of blindness, possessed and generated by individuals with sight, can lead to low expectations which service providers sometimes have for those whom they serve (Koestler 1976: 7) and to sentimental pity or sympathy prompted by even the most superficial contact (Monbeck 1973: 4). Indeed, there is little doubt that the misconceptions of the sighted have a disturbing impact on the visually-impaired person's sense of her/himself. Robert Scott notes:

> blindness is a stigma, carrying with it a series of moral
> imputations about character and personality. The stereotypical
> beliefs . . . lead normal people to feel that the blind are

different; the fact that blindness is a stigma leads them to regard the blind men as their physical, psychological, moral and emotional inferiors. Blindness is therefore a trait that discredits a man by spoiling both his identity and his respectability. (1969: 24)

It is therefore quite understandable that many contemporary writers about blindness seek to minimize the costs of blindness and vision loss, to the point of almost denying its delimiting effects. A prototypical instance of this tendency can be found in Kenneth Jernigan's (1965) attempt to describe blindness in neutral terms. He insists that it is a 'characteristic' rather than a 'handicap.' As leader of the National Federation of the Blind – an active consumer-advocacy group – Jernigan's interest in replacing the negative meaning of 'handicap' with the less judgemental term 'characteristic' is perfectly understandable and makes sound political sense. It also assists the process of consciousness-raising that is so important to social movements of any sort. But do such semantic changes make experiential sense? Does 'characteristic' capture the experience of vision loss? While such treatments of vision loss may be helpful in avoiding numerous aspects of the stigma so often attached to this sensory loss, they serve to foster still other misconceptions about the losses and limitations so clearly perceived by visually-impaired actors themselves. For the person experiencing new vision loss late in life, it is precisely the misconceptions of the sighted world that make their apprehension so great, and their anxieties as well as fears are all too real. This leads one to ask 'Whose reality is at issue?'

The effects of new vision loss on one's daily life are among the most central preoccupations of the person who is adventitiously visually impaired. In their actual daily experience, the ideological concerns of persons with blindness, conceived as a group too long disparaged by the larger society, give way to the day-to-day concerns with previously-taken-for-granted activities which are now an unending series of problematic situations.

In the judgement of one 83 year old, new vision loss is 'a son of a gun thing. You have to give up all activity practically. You can't do anything. And ah, I would say that it is one of the worst things that can happen to you outside of cancer.' For this individual, new vision loss is no mere characteristic among others. It rather carries with it a continual stream of challenges to those things which he once did without the slightest thought. In Alfred Schutz's (1971) terms, he has lost his past 'familiarity' with the world, i.e. it may be difficult for him readily to place the new experiences accompanying his vision loss into what Schutz terms the 'stock of already acquired knowledge.'

Throughout their lives, people accumulate information about themselves, others, and the world around them. Much of this information is passed on by predecessors (family, teachers, and others) through the process of socialization. Hence an individual is born into a world that is, as Schutz also observes, already 'shot through meaning.' Predecessors pass on to their biological and social heirs tried interpretations of experience, which then become critical to the successors' participation in the world. To these tried interpretations, the individual then adds new ones as experiences arise which are not easily handled by existing information. Much of growing up is a matter of modifying and adding to this accumulated stock of knowledge. The individual's familiarity with the world is tied to the adequacy of this stock of knowledge. For the individual who has spent the first fifty or sixty years of her/his life relying on visual cues to order their activities, the loss of sight calls for more than slight modifications in both their interpretations and their lifestyle.

Even the most elementary skills involved in eating, for example, can become problematic without the visual cues upon which a person has traditionally relied.

> I go over there to eat at the senior citizens center and I don't know the person next to me until I get used to them. That is, to their voice. I can't see their faces and, ah, well, I'm clumsy in eating. There are times when I don't know if I'm going to stick my god damn fork in my mouth or in my ear.

Another 77 year old echoes this report.

> If someone didn't cut the food on my plate, I couldn't eat.
> When I'm alone to eat, I'll pour the water for my coffee next to the cup. Or if I want to take a glass of water, instead of grabbing it I just knock it off. I just don't see it.

Nearly every person had a story of spilled drinks, misplaced hands in foods, uncertainties about table settings, etc. These problems with eating, however, signal only a small part of the overall delimiting impact new vision loss has on the life of the person confronted for the first time with the loss of such a taken-for-granted sensory tool.

With the loss of sight one's immediate physical environment, through which the person used to navigate with ease, now becomes a sort of obstacle course. One person described, for example, her encounter with the furniture in her home: 'You have to remember where you put things, like I said. I often stub my toe on chairs and when I stoop over to grab my toe, I bang my head.' Jacob Van Weelden (1967) observes that people may develop a 'hostile' relationship with the physical objects in their environment. He notes that 'buckets left in a corridor, doors standing half open, overhanging branches, awnings are loathed by every blind person – to the blind person bending down the back of a chair may prove itself particularly malicious' (1967: 42). Almost as if recalling a joke told in poor taste – but illustrating Van Weelden's point – another person spoke of the perils of his wife's weekly cleaning efforts.

She used to move the furniture when she would house clean. She would move the furniture all around and it would take a couple of days to get used to it again. You know? I would keep bumping into the coffee table or something like that.

The obstacles of the home are often put in order with the cooperative efforts of the other members of the household. Nevertheless, there are always times when the necessarily constant attention to the placement of furniture and other even more movable articles wanes. In these instances persons who are visually impaired soon realize their dependence upon order, and their vulnerability to changes in their environment.

Every person had a full catalog of activities which proved difficult, if not seemingly impossible, to master. At almost every turn of their daily agenda, they struggled with one of a variety of new challenges posed by their sensory limitation. It doesn't take a special occasion or particularly unusual activity to remind the person experiencing vision loss of her/his new way of life. As one lay-phenomenologist describes it:

It is the little everyday things that you did and you took for granted. Those are the things. Those are the things that bother me more than anything else. It's those little things that you go to do that you don't even think about ordinarily that create the biggest problems. I blow them all out of proportion, you know?

One of the more notable of the daily activities drastically curtailed by vision loss is the ability to read. Magazines, newspapers, books, directions on the back of various food items, recipes, etc., all become indecipherable in severe cases of vision loss. Even for those persons who retain some usable eyesight, the task may be so painstaking as to discourage its undertaking. An individual with some remaining vision describes the slow process of digesting the printed word.

I can't say I enjoy reading because I can't read that much. I
have low vision glasses but I still don't see what I want. You
know? I mean, normally a person speed reads more. I never
was one to read one word and then move on and this kills me.

Under normal circumstances, a person takes in a sentence as a
whole, placing each word within the context of the others. For
persons with a visual impairment, each word (sometimes each
letter) must be taken by itself, and some report that by the time
they reach the final word of a sentence, they have forgotten those
at its beginning. This difficulty with reading and the corresponding
problems associated with writing make written communication
with the outside world quite difficult. For those who are unable to
make out even the single word, the problem is even more
fundamental. With only three weeks remaining before Christmas,
another person lamented her inability (for the first time) to write
greeting cards as she had done for each of the preceding fifty-three
years.

I'm not going to have any Christmas this year. I bought a box of
Christmas cards but I just can't see to write or address them.
Yesterday it took me all afternoon to address just one
envelope. And that I got all crooked. I couldn't spell it right
either. So I tore it up and tried another one. But my eyes – a
year ago I could write letters and cards pretty good, but now
there's no hope for me.

As will be suggested in the next chapter, the inability to
correspond through the written word is an important dimension of
the constrictions in one's contact with the social world, as well as
one of the early signs to the individual of her/his own biological
decline.

Of course there are a myriad of other activities in one's daily life
which were once part of the general background of taken-for-
granted tasks which now are all too apparent as hindrances.

I can't tell the knobs on my stove, you know, the temperature. I
have an awful time with that and of course on my washing
machine they had to put tape so I can see the cycles. I made a
mess of that for a long time. They put masking tape on the
normal cycle and another tape on the gentle cycle and I feel it
with my hands, you know? That's how I see. I can't see the
clock. I can't tell time unless I take the clock in my hands. I
can't sew or crochet or knit or embroider and things like that. I
have to try and feel if I want to iron. When I want to watch TV,
I put my face up as close as I possibly can to it and then all I get

is the words, you know? I can't cook. I can't peel potatoes. I'm just as likely to boil the peelings and throw the potatoes away. Well, it may sound silly but that's the way it is.

The disruptions of daily activities and the difficulties of navigating through personal artifacts force the person to focus inordinately upon activities that were previously taken for granted. Except when prompted to think about it, people do not think about the way they read a sentence, the way they locate an empty table in a restaurant, the way they maneuver through a living room. They simply take these skills, these activities, for granted. New vision loss represents a severe instance, then, of those problematic situations which from time to time challenge people's hold of the world. In principle, it parallels Schutz and Luckmann's (1973: 103) discussion of a pulled tooth. As they describe the experience, people are at first fascinated and preoccupied with the hole in their mouth. They continually touch the spot with their tongue. The tooth's absence 'brings into relief' the normally taken-for-granted experience people have of their mouths. Of course, the contrast with the routine functioning of the body is greater with new vision loss than with the loss of a tooth. The taken for granted is brought into relief to a much greater degree. Similarly, however, it brings the normally-background assumptions to the center stage of action in and upon the world.

Navigating the home surely presents a number of problems, but the outside world, which remains unimpressed with the need for order, presents an unending array of obstacles as well. Each step down a sidewalk takes on an air of uncertainty and each curb threatens a fall, such that older persons experiencing new vision loss are often tentative and on their guard.

When I go downtown, well, if there's a little bump on the sidewalk or something like that, I trip over it. If I come to a curb, well, sometimes I miss one. So even though I was born and brought up in this area, in this section of town, I seldom go out alone. Never at night. I did once and had a hard time to come back. As a rule, I never go out alone.

Accepting stereotypical notions about the resiliency of youth long since passed and the limitations of their age, many of the people expressed fears of falling, fears of injury to themselves in a world which they no longer see well enough to feel competent to manipulate. Unfortunately, their fear of their physical vulnerability is often confirmed by near misses and actual injuries. Several people explained their reluctance to go beyond the confines of their own home by recalling incidents which made this vulnerability all too plain.

> I can't go no further than the yard here. I don't even dare to cross the street. One day last summer, I wanted to go down the street where they [city employees] were working on a water pump. Down below here by the river. I was in the corner of my lot here and thought everything was quiet. I couldn't see any cars coming so I started to cross the road. By Jesus, there was a motorcycle coming that went right by me. Just missed me. Oh Jesus! That's the last time I been across the road. So you see what I mean? I don't dare go across the street.

Others were not so fortunate. Several had actually been struck by cars. Although not seriously injured, it was enough to dissuade them from traveling any distance alone. The hostility of the objects around them was again confirmed.

As residents in most communities without elaborate mass transportation will attest, the inability to drive a car represents one of the most staggering of setbacks. It is almost essential to be able to drive in order to secure subsistence goods and to fulfill social obligations. As such, the inability to drive which follows the loss of vision is often hard to bear.

> I had to get rid of my car. Why, I felt like jumping off a bridge. We had a nice car we liked an awful lot. An Oldsmobile. But what the hell is the use of having a car if you can't use it? And of course I couldn't go back to get my license. I wouldn't think of going back. Wouldn't get it anyway. And boy, that was pretty tough on me. Now if I want to go somewhere I have to call somebody.

Many people admit that they drove their cars long after they should have, given the amount of remaining sight they possessed. In several cases, it took an accident to convince them that they would have to give it up.

> The last time I drove a car I ran into a little squall and lost the road completely. I went right through a telephone post and just sat there parked. Fortunately, the person coming the other direction knew me and my condition. He came up and said 'Are you all right?' and I says 'Yeah, I'm all right but this is the last time I'm going to drive my car.' He called my son to come and get me and that was it.

The reluctance of people to give up driving, even at some personal risk, is certainly evidence of the automobile's import as a means of accessing the distant physical environment. It also seemed, however, that the automobile represented another symbol of normalcy which people found particularly difficult to sacrifice.

The worry about injury, the inability to drive, the problems of personal mobility, all tend to reduce a person's willingness and capacity to carry on many of the activities outside the home which once simply represented an imposition on her/his time. Now these activities not only take more time but serve to remind the person all too well of her/his visual difficulties and prove a source of tremendous frustration. Many cited the shopping experience, in particular, as one of the most troubling. Whereas in the past they were able to run in and out of a store to pick up a needed item, with the advent of vision loss they found that the selection of goods could be a grueling affair.

> It's really maddening at times. But what bothers me is to go in –
> when I want to buy something at the store: clothing or
> something like that – and I can't see the prices or anything else.
> You know that just means that you have to ask somebody at
> your side or take it to one of the clerks to ask them if they'll
> please tell you what size something is or what the price is. Of
> course, for several years now I haven't been able to take
> something off the shelves – like in a grocery store – and tell
> what the price is. So you just have to make up your mind that
> you will take it regardless of the price. Sometimes this can be
> very embarrassing because many times there is not a clerk
> around and you have to ask another customer if they would
> mind telling you. Perhaps one out of ten just walks away from
> you and that kind of cuts.

As indicated by this person's remarks, it is quite common for persons with vision loss to avoid (if at all possible) the problems they know to be associated with their vision loss. In the above-cited case, this individual would rather take an item not knowing its cost rather than risk the embarrassment of asking for assistance.

Without the ability to confirm visually the course of her/his actions, the experience of new vision loss often presents the individual with unanticipated consequences. One person told of waiting for friends who were going to drive her to a dinner engagement and the series of events which followed.

> I was waiting for friends to come get me. At the same time a
> neighbor lady next to me was expecting someone to pick her up
> too. Well, this car outside toots its horn, you know? I go out,
> get in the car and I sit down. Well, I got into the wrong car!

Thank God I knew the people. So they started teasing me. They said 'Well, we're going out to play bingo and you're welcome to come along with us.' I said 'No, but thank you. I've got into the wrong car.' I got out of that car and the neighbor woman came up. I said 'This is your car. It's not mine.' Well, I didn't even have time to get back up to the house when my friends drove up. I got in and I said 'Oh, I feel so foolish.' You feel like a fool but these things will happen.

Other people had their own stories of situations which emerged from their inability to confirm their intentions visually. Several complained of going to restrooms at restaurants, only to return to the wrong table. Others told of becoming totally disoriented in a public place, such as a shopping mall, and having to wait until friends noticed their plight. Such experiences not only remind visually-impaired persons of their susceptibility to error, but discourage the very undertaking of activities they would otherwise seek out. One 60 year old, whose husband had died some three years earlier, spoke of her reluctance to follow the encouragement of her friends to go out and meet new people.

If there's something I don't think I can handle I won't go out. I won't put myself in that spot, you know, not to be accepted. If I feel there is the slightest doubt I won't go. I'll stay home. Avoid this. Like going out dancing. My greatest fear was that I'd go and I'd go dancing and then I'd have to get back to my table. Of course the man is supposed to take you back to your table but I'd say to myself 'What if he meets somebody and starts talking?' I'd think 'I'd feel foolish with all those people around.'

Not only, then, is the person's confidence in her/his ability to manipulate the world shaken, but a certain propensity toward social isolation is encouraged (which will be addressed more fully in the chapter to follow).

The inability to confirm the environment, which for a person with sight may take only a single glance, constantly confronts persons with vision loss. Precisely because they traditionally took this capacity to confirm visually their intentions for granted, they frequently find themselves committed to a course of action which requires sight only to realize (too late) that they no longer can visually orient themselves in the world.

It is also important to recognize that the limitations upon activity imposed by new vision loss are often compounded by other physical factors. Some of these may be related to the vision problem itself. Diabetes, for example, often carries with it other serious physical problems. In severe instances, it may be necessary for legs to be amputated, which not only adds to the already problematic nature of mobility but also makes it seem to people that their bodies are 'giving out' all at once. One person interviewed, for example, had become legally blind, lost one of her legs, and was threatened with the loss of the other – all within one year's time. Each loss afforded her undeniable evidence of her physical decline.

Most compounding factors are, however, more characteristic of the process of aging in more general terms. People complained of diverticulitis, muscular disorders, back problems, and the loss of other sensory skills (most notably hearing). Each of these conditions usually required a host of medications and only magnified the already tentative nature of people's embrace of the world around them. These compounding physical factors affect much of the aging population for which they are suggestive of the inevitable biological decline that accompanies old age. For persons with new visual impairment, these additional physical concerns increase their preoccupation with the personal fallibility they already experience because of the loss of their eyesight.

Changing recipe knowledge

The curtailment of activities brought on by age-related visual impairments challenges the very interpretive categories by which people's knowledge of their bodies and the world around them is ordered. Bestowing meaning on the world – which again is part of everyone's ongoing effort to make sense of her/his life – is made possible by what phenomenologists term 'recipes.' These recipes, or the 'repertoires of rules people possess for handling and manipulating things and events' (Gurwitsch 1974: 118), are taken for granted by most people. For the person approaching old age, these recipes are often challenged by new and unfamiliar situations of all kinds. Of particular relevance are the assorted novel situations that are prompted by the biological decline of the aging organism. From the discussion above it should be quite clear that age-related vision loss challenges the existing recipes of the older person in a number of notable ways.

It has already been demonstrated that, in terms of the actors themselves, new vision loss is not a mere characteristic among others. Rather, as Francis Dover observes, 'the onset of blindness is certainly a severe blow to the total person, shaking to the core his previous life adjustment' (1959: 334). A person doesn't have visual impairments in the way another person may have freckles.

New vision loss challenges people's very hold on their physical environment, their bodies, and, as will be ultimately demonstrated, their hold on their sense of self. The difficulties in eating one's own food, the propensity towards spilling drinks, the constant threat of injury from furniture, cracks in the pavement, garbage cans, bicycles, etc., the loss of independent access to far-off places, the difficulties in reading and writing, as well as the host of situations which require sight to implement intentions successfully – all these things surely force people to re-examine taken-for-granted life upon which they can no longer depend.

In Edmund Husserl's terms, the disruption of one's life as it was taken for granted when the person possessed a full range of visual skills has a disruptive impact upon the 'I-can-do-it-again' idealization. As Schutz summarizes this idealization, it is the 'assumption that I may under typically similar circumstances act in a way typically similar to that in which I acted before in order to bring about a typically similar state of affairs' (1971: 20). In other words, a person can impose a certain order on the world simply by believing that what has been accomplished before can be accomplished again, given similar circumstances. This belief is, of course, challenged by new vision loss. Without the visual skills typically used to guide their actions, people can no longer assume that actions will unfold in the same way as they did before they developed problems with their sight. On the contrary, their day-to-day experiences constantly remind them of the problems associated with their attempts to carry on as usual.

Like anyone else, persons who are visually impaired attempt to force their new life back into the unproblematic. Peter Berger and Thomas Luckmann (1966: 24) give the example of an automobile mechanic who routinely works on American cars and who, for the first time, confronts a Volkswagen. In such a moment, routine experience becomes questionable. It must be examined and hopefully integrated into the unproblematic. Just as the automobile mechanic attempts to integrate the repair of a Volkswagen into the unproblematic – discovering that despite differences there are enough similarities to proceed – persons experiencing vision loss try to restore their lives to the routine. Because they no longer can rely on their once-taken-for-granted visual skills and because the world around them is by and large organized by the sighted, their attempts to restore their lives into the routine are constantly frustrated.

> If you don't remember where you put a tool or if you kick a tool around or if you accidentally move anything around, you are

lost. Even here at home, if my wife moves my stuff around then I am lost. If she doesn't put the milk in the refrigerator always in the same place, or the juice, then I have to start hunting and I get my hands in the wrong kind of dishes. You often knock stuff down, you know?

What was once accomplished with ease can now become an ordeal, and as such the attempts to carry on as usual often require slow and methodical attention.

I was a big worker all of my life. . . . I was always doing something. I'm still a pusher. I want to do this, do that, do this, do that. But now I can't always do it. I still try to do all my own work. I used to clean this whole room in one day. Now I can't do it. I can't do it. I just can't. Your whole body just seems to slow down.

Despite the frustrations which evolve from the failures to accomplish what the person intends and the now painstaking efforts required to achieve goals, for many the attempts to integrate their new life into the unproblematic becomes their *raison d'être*.

Well now it takes me, oh a week to do what I used to do in a day. You know? So it is different. At the very first I was much less active than I had been because I was so discouraged. I thought I couldn't do anything if I couldn't see, you know? I mean it was really hard to do things and so many things would come up during the day that I couldn't do because I couldn't see to do it. So at the beginning it is really frustrating, of course. You really have to learn to do things all over again. And so I couldn't be as active. But there didn't seem to be any other way so I just felt that if I was going to live then I had to do it. Because I just couldn't sit around and not have it done. It would drive me crazy just to sit.

The success they have at reapproaching the routine seems to derive mostly from their rigorous ordering of their environment. Careful placement of objects in their near surroundings and attention to organizational detail facilitates the ordering process. But this ordering remains precarious. When the order is breached (by the person her/himself or by others) or when they find themselves in unfamiliar settings, they become acutely aware of the fact that the routine will be constantly challenged.

The efforts required for the person to come to grips with the new recipes of this new life seemingly take their toll. In the words of one person, the loss of eyesight seemed to mark the turning point of his very sense of himself as 'old.' Until he began losing his sight he felt like he was in fairly good physical condition and maintained an active schedule. With his vision loss, however,

> Well things changed. I feel I've gotten much older. I can tell you that. It's because of this problem – that I don't see. This has made me feel older. I was not feeling old before. I was healthy enough for my age, you know? But this – this has gotten me.

He reported that this change in his perception of himself as old was, in part, produced by the increased weariness he felt. Others commonly confirmed this feeling of tiredness and attributed it to the demanding nature of attempts to adapt to limited visual abilities.

> I go to bed at night and I sleep. 'Cause I've been active all day. I go to bed exhausted at night. I say 'My God! I've had a busy day.' You know? 'Cause before things were so easy. Like if you needed a phone number, you'd just pick up the phone book and look it up. But now, if you want a number, well you say 'What is it?' and you wait until it pops up in your mind. But you've really got to think of it to remember. You have to notice things a lot more. 'Cause before, you'd just look and that was it. Everything was a lot easier before.

The organization of space and time

The ability of the aging person experiencing new vision loss to act upon space can be drastically curtailed. All the senses can play important roles in the subjective determination of one's location in space (although some argue that taste might be excluded; see Van Weelden 1967). Those which serve as receptors of distant information (the eyes, ears, and nose) are perhaps most obviously central to spatial experience. Yet even the skin has been shown to be instrumental to subjective self-placement through detection and emission of radiant heat (Hall 1966: 54ff.). Of the senses, however, it is sight that provides the individual with the most information about space – especially distant space. The loss of sight therefore curtails the individual's ability to gather much of the sensory information by which her/his spatial relations with other objects, artifacts, written word, and other people are established. In a word, it makes space problematic.

> It is particularly troubling because you are used to using your eyes all the time and when you can't you have got to feel your

way around. It is sometimes very frustrating. For instance when
you look for something on the floor. When you see well you just
see it. But when your eyes are gone, well it might have rolled
five or six feet away. So what you used to do in a couple of
seconds may sometimes take you five or six minutes to try and
find it. You expect things like that.

Or as another person reported,

Even in the house you have to put things in the same place
'cause if you don't you can go hunting around for different
things for hours. Like my glasses. I used to just put them in the
same spot all the time so I will know where to get them when I
need them. I have done a lot of hunting around for different
things I've lost.

As Van Weelden observes, 'objects often hide themselves from
being observed by the blind so that they are unknowable. Things
which can only be perceived visually are "invisible"' (1967: 38).
Only those things which can be committed to memory or
confirmed by tactile observation can also be spatially placed.
Those things which are forgotten no longer have spatial meaning
until they are recalled or rediscovered through non-visual means.
   Most newly-visually-impaired persons have some remaining
vision and as such the world around them still provides some visual
information. This remaining world of visual clues is often
described as a 'haze' or 'fog' or continuous 'blur,' only occasionally
broken by movement or color. This world which lacks visual
clarity can actually provide the person with inaccurate information
about the spatial arrangements of objects and indeed the objects
themselves.

Sometimes you'll see something is there but you don't know if
it's something that's standing up or laying down. You don't
know if it's a shadow or a hole. You can't tell. I'll see a shadow
and sometimes I don't know if it's something in my way or not.
You know? Or sometimes there will be a patch in the sidewalk
or a patch in the road which seems darker.

On occasion this confusion in visual clues leads the person to
conclude that 'Sometimes I think it would be easier with no sight at
all than just a little bit of sight because you still depend on your
sight and that throws you off.' Thus, not only are some objects
which surround the visually-impaired person unknowable, but
those which remain available to persons with some limited vision
are subject to error. Action in and upon space therefore often

becomes a matter of faith in the way things were or in the way they seem. Of course, everyone is tied to her/his own perspectival hold on space but for the person with visual impairment this hold is often challenged by frequent confrontations with an organization of space which contradicts her/his faithful renderings.

When the person's organization of spatial arrangements is challenged or contradicted, a certain sense of 'disorientation' seems to predominate. In Lofland's terms, disorientation is 'precipitated by the occurrence of events that fall outside or between actor's existing cognitive categories for rendering reality coherent and understandable' (1969: 178). As one person noted,

> You are afraid. . . . A person that loses their sight – you are completely disoriented because you no longer have any sense of direction. Like a hunter in the woods who is lost – he might be walking around in circles so that he actually stays in the same place when he thinks he is going out of the woods. A blind person is like that too.

In an effort to insure that this sort of disorientation is minimized, people who are losing their sight are often counseled to familiarize themselves with their environment in anticipation of further vision losses.

> I go around the house [with the lights out] and I make sure I feel my way around in the dark to see how it would be. I will be all right if nobody moves the furniture or something like that. I do this a lot – I pretend that I'm completely blind and go around.

Chairs normally considered to facilitate comfort now threaten injury; areas through which one once moved unthinkingly must now be carefully studied and committed to memory. In effect, people are asked to relearn the space around them in ways which minimize their dependence upon its visual signals.

People soon learn that vision loss carries with it a well-developed battery of 'hardware' by which they can learn to navigate through their environment. Lofland defines hardware as 'those physical objects that can be affixed to the body of an actor and those that can be picked up or manipulated' (1969: 174). All people use hardware to some degree to extend their bodily manipulation of the space around them. As has already been seen, some of the normal hardware of daily life, such as automobiles, are withdrawn from people experiencing new severe vision loss. In their place are other extensions of their body which ultimately become the very symbols of their abnormality. Most notable in this regard is the white cane. Many people reported that coming to terms with such symbols of abnormality was one of the more difficult aspects of their adaptation to vision loss.

> Well, when I took mobility lessons – I think that was the hardest thing I ever did in my life. It was for me. To go down the street where everyone knows you, you know? With a cane. That was hard.

Other pieces of hardware are often readily apparent when one enters the home of persons with severe visual impairment. Large-print books and magazines, canes in the corners of rooms, cases with recorded books, and the usual host of magnifying devices, betray the person's struggle to adjust as well as the usually well-meant intervention of family, friends, and service providers.

Not only is the sense of space altered with new vision loss but so too is the perception of time – the individual's sense of a present sandwiched between past and future (I use time here in a somewhat limited sense – not to refer to socio-historical location in a more macro sense). The world is experienced in terms of the relative closeness and remoteness to the present, and it is the present which looms so important when visual skills are called into question.

> When you are starting to lose your sight there are a lot of things that you appreciate more than if you had your sight. There are a lot of things that you normally don't look at or take the time to look at and enjoy. You know? Like if it's a beautiful day, you don't just enjoy it. But if you lose your sight, you enjoy it. You go out and you say 'oh, it's a beautiful day.' I guess in the back of your mind you think 'Well, gee, if I should go totally blind at least I've seen this or I've done that.' You know? You appreciate things more. You notice things more.

The person losing her/his sight places a high priority, then, on what Schutz (1971) calls the 'vivid present' or the 'just now.' The present, for all people, becomes meaningful only in its connection to the past in the person's recollections and to the future in the person's anticipations. The individual experiencing vision loss, however, embraces the vivid present in an effort to hold on to the fleeting recollections of the past.

> It [vision loss] has made me appreciate some of the things that you take for granted. With not being able to see you appreciate what was ordinarily, I mean, what was just an accepted thing. I missed a lot of the beauty of the fall foliage this year because I don't see much. There was a lot of the beauty that I couldn't get

but I remember the beauty that has been here for so long and I appreciate what I could still see this year, you know?

Furthermore, people long to hold on to the vivid present because they cannot be sure of what the future will bring. 'It's a new chapter, you know? Before I could live for tomorrow and say "Well, tomorrow we'll do this" or "the next day we'll do something else." No more.' Because they are uncertain about the future progression of their vision loss, and because they are reluctant to give up the visual world they once took for granted, people embrace the present with apparent intensity.

Back and Gergen (1968) have noted that with declines in people's sense of bodily well-being there is a corresponding constriction in 'life/space extensity.' This is to suggest that in the face of the decline in the biological organism, aging persons begin to doubt their ability to act upon both time and space. The result is that people place a low priority on affecting changes in their physical environment and are reluctant to dwell upon anticipations of future events. This should be apparent from the immediately preceding quote. People addressed this issue in greater detail when responding to queries about their plans for the future. One suggested, for example,

I don't make any plans. I don't hope for anything. I'm just living from day to day. I never plan ahead or hope to do this or hope to do that. No, I never plan. I never do that. Today I'm here and tomorrow – well tomorrow I may be in the hospital or somewhere else. I just don't know.

By their own estimates, this is the only reasonable response to their circumstance. 'I know I can't reach my goals, I just can't reach those points. So I take life as it comes.' With philosophical resolve, many people report that they would rather focus upon what can be done at present with their remaining vision than be preoccupied with a future full of uncertainty.

I just go from one day to the next. I just want to do the best I can with every day. I don't really have any special goals. I think maybe it's because I don't know just how bad my sight will get. And maybe I'm kind of thinking that I'll want a certain goal and I won't be able to do it. I don't want to try to do too much, you know? Something I can't handle. So I think it's better if I just take it day to day and live each day to the fullest. Not planning too far ahead, you know?

Both the time and the space considered relevant are mediated by their sense of their own newly-limited corporeal being.

Reactions to new vision loss

There is remarkable consistency in the informants' accountings of the impact of sensory decline upon their day-to-day activities, their recipes for actions in the world, and their perceptions of both space and time. Yet in their reactions to the impact of new vision loss, persons do not always apply the same interpretations such that, while there are common reactions to sensory loss, not everyone experiences all of them nor do they exhibit them to the same degree or in the same order of appearance. While many writers in studies of blindness have attempted to discuss the typical stages of adjustment to vision loss (see Bauman 1954, Dover 1959, Freedman 1965, Adams and Pearlman 1970, Altshuler 1970, Fitzgerald 1971, Kirtley 1975), it is very clear that, in the actual experience of new vision loss, Dover (1959: 337) is correct in observing not every person goes through all the various stages outlined. As she puts it, 'all these reactions can be experienced simultaneously, partially, one at a time or in different combinations.' They may also be experienced in varying degrees of intensity. Therefore, it is inappropriate to speak of predictable stages of adjustment to vision loss. Nevertheless, it is possible to catalog some of the common reactions exhibited by persons facing new vision loss and to begin to place them in an experiential context.

One initial reaction to vision loss which was almost universally reported was the feeling of disbelief. While many people have to wear glasses for most of their lives – usually to compensate for one of the near-universal changes in the eye with age – few have any reason to believe that their respective minor exposures to myopia or astigmatism will eventually give way to severe visual disorders. One person recalled the initial diagnosis of glaucoma.

> I never really had any problems with my eyes. I wore glasses. I was farsighted so I'd wear them to see up close, for reading, you know? But I never, never had any real problems. Never. I never expected to lose my sight. Never. That's why when the doctor told me I had glaucoma, I was so surprised. I didn't have headaches. I had nothing to show for it. I had gone in for my annual checkup and he was changing my lenses. Then he said 'I think that we'll check the pressure.' When he did the pressure was way, way up and all. At first I couldn't believe it. I said, 'my gosh, I've no headaches.' You expect those, I guess. They tell you you're supposed to see halos around lights. But I didn't have headaches – nothing at all. No symptoms at all.

Of course, for most people the signs of vision loss usually become apparent before the problem is confirmed by ophthalmological examinations. The disbelief is nevertheless apparent here as well.

Well, it's something that you cannot believe is happening to you to start with. They tell you you got good vision and then you get this thing and you say 'Oh no! I can't believe it!' You know? You can't believe you'll lose your eyesight. You just won't believe it.

As was suggested earlier, the realization that one is actually experiencing severe vision loss can be postponed at least for a while. Many people reported that they had tried at first to explain away their vision difficulties – tired eyes, the need for lens changes, high blood pressure, or any of a variety of other readily-available alternative explanations. Eventually, however, persons were persuaded by the persistence of visual difficulties to seek out professional evaluations. They often hoped until the last possible moment that some corrective procedure would somehow allow them to avoid the inevitable.

When the doctor examined me and told me [there was nothing he could do] I could have gone through the floor. I came out and I think I was actually numb. I lost all concept of everything. I mean, I just felt like that was it. Well, it was just like he said 'You're legally blind.' If there had been a hole I think I would have gone right down – clear all the way down. That was it. That was the end of the line. I think it was just the impact. Because I was a positive thinking person, I figure he was going to tell me that they could do something. They'd shoot a laser beam or they could operate or they could do something.

Again, for some people there are medical or surgical remedies which afford them comfort. The pressure of glaucoma can be controlled, some cataracts can be removed, etc. These remedies can often enable individuals to stabilize their visual condition or at least retard the progression of visual losses. Those, for whom medical and surgical remedies remain even a marginal possibility, are buoyed by the hope that this gives them. A person with glaucoma, for instance, observed

I keep thinking 'Oh, maybe I'll get better, maybe I'll get better eyesight.' You know? I think people do that. They just keep thinking it will get better. I think that's what keeps us going. 'Cause if we kept thinking it's only going to get worse and what it could turn into – I mean, you can't live with something like that. I keep thinking maybe it will get better.

Those for whom there are no medical or surgical remedies gradually come to realize that there is little they can do to ignore the decline of their aging body. They often feel a resulting sense of disorientation or dislocation. The disruption of their life-course posed by sensory decline seems to leave them puzzled about both present and future.

I started to lose my vision about five years ago. So I went to see different doctors and specialists here in town. They said it was hardening of the arteries. They said there was nothing that I could do about it. There's no medication or no operation whatsoever. Now five years later, I have lost the sight in one eye. The doctor says, 'Well, after all, your age is there.' So what can you do when they tell you your age is there? What are you going to do?

Sometimes this sense of dislocation gives way to panic.

Well, at first you think it can't be true. You won't accept it, you know? Like it can't be happening to me. And then, well you kind of get panicky. You'll cry. And then you try everything out. You pray a lot. You keep hoping that a miracle will happen. That you will see again. It must be the same with everything. Like if you lose a leg, I imagine people go through the same thing, you know? They probably also get panicky and say 'this can't be happening to me.' When you can't do anything about it and you keep getting worse – if there's an operation or some help you can get well, I suppose it's different. When there's nothing to be done, it really scares you.

Sometimes, then, the disbelief that

1 it is happening to them and
2 that there is nothing that can be done

leads people to seek out other options and a variety of therapies. Several individuals told of going to five or more specialists in the hopes that a different doctor might provide a different diagnosis or prognosis. Most maintained that they would have tried almost any remedy had such been forthcoming. This has been confirmed in other studies. Fitzgerald's (1971) study of newly-blind persons in London, for example, reported that 35 per cent of his sample had gone to faith healers once they had exhausted more orthodox treatments. Andrew Potok's (1980) autobiographical account of new vision loss further confirms the lengths to which the disbelief at one's own plight can carry the person. Potok exposed himself for weeks to painful bee-sting 'therapy' in the hope of a miracle cure. While none of the people that I talked with availed themselves of these sorts of remedies, their disbelief at their own sensory fallibility and the ineffectiveness of modern medical techniques often revealed their susceptibility to both orthodox and unorthodox solutions to their visual demise.

Many people face the continuing day-to-day reminders of their vision loss with a certain anger. After many daily confrontations with the obstacles that his vision loss placed in the way of his daily agenda, one person spoke of the anger he now felt toward his own ineptness.

> I can't seem to stand what I used to stand. I can't do a god-damned thing right. I once was considered one of the best craftsmen in my trade. But I can't do anything right today. I don't care what I try to tackle, it's wrong. Now I get ugly awfully easy. Yeah, now I get mad at myself. I do foolish things, you know? Like knocking down things on to something. I says 'You goddamned idiot, stupid son of a bitch.' You know? I don't know what the hell you'd call that 'cept ugly. I'd say I get mad easy, let's put it that way.

Not all the anger is directed by the person with visual impairments toward her/himself. As Dover has noted from her own studies, 'frequently the newly blind person directs his anger toward and attributes his handicap to the incompetence of the physician in charge of his case' (1959: 336). While many visually-impaired persons show anger for themselves, they often have plenty in reserve for the medical profession.

> I went to see an ophthalmologist in Maine. See, I had lost my driver's license and so I says to him 'I'd like to get my eye fixed up enough so that I could get my license back again.' Well, he says, 'I'll fix you up.' And I says 'Well, that's all I expect.' Well, instead of fixing me up – he blinded me. I lost my eyesight altogether. And besides that, I had given him over eight hundred dollars. Well, he called me later and still wanted some four hundred dollars or so more. I says 'Well, you bastards, you just try and get it.' I wish they'd sue me for it because I'd use every cent I've got to fight them. I haven't got much but I hate to be taken for a sucker, you know? I don't mind spending a dollar but I hate to be cheated out of a nickel.

Anger, especially toward oneself and the inability to do things one once did, is reportedly experienced to some degree by most people in the early months of visual impairment (see Dover 1959). It seems difficult to maintain the intensity of this anger over the years. Nevertheless, several people harbored this reaction as long as seven to ten years after the onset of severe vision loss. Others seemed to extend their anger toward members of the medical profession involved in their treatment for nearly as long.

As the realization that visual impairment was now a permanent part of their life began to sink in, many people reported a fear of what their reduced visual capacity would bring. One individual, after being thoroughly tested and retested and finally told that she had retinitis pigmentosa, reported that her thoughts were with

> jumping out the window and you know we were eleven stories up. The first night was terrible, a terrible night. I guess it's just everything because you don't think you will be able to cope with everyday life. I was just frantic because I didn't think I would be able to do my housework, take care of my home, my clothes – everything you have to do in everyday life. Everything. You just don't think you can do it. I just didn't see how I was going to live and not see.

This person betrays the ultimate frustration reported by Chevigny (1946), i.e. 'being unable even to commit suicide without help.'

Another individual, upon learning of his retinal detachment, reported

> There is a great fear because you say to yourself 'Well, when I don't see no more that will be the end of the world.' It's true, too, when you have always done things for yourself and you find now you can't do things like that. It's like that for everybody, I guess.

Thus, the anticipated discontinuity between people's previously-sighted and now visually-impaired lives prompts fear, puzzlement, and in some case panic at the uncertain future life will bring.

The initial reactions to the pronouncement of their present or impending visual condition is, of course, linked to the preconceptions that individuals developed as sighted actors. While it is easy to discount the misconceptions of persons with sight toward persons with blindness from the stance of scientific observer, it is impossible to do so in accounting for the experience of a new visual impairment. Assurances such as 'you can continue to live a full life' or 'blindness is only a characteristic' cannot dissipate the years of stereotypical preconceptions and now-lived experience of the very real difficulties imposed by new vision loss. Thus, the grooves and channels into which the sighted place their expectations for people with blindness (helplessness, docility, dependency, melancholia, aestheticism, and serious-mindedness, to

51

mention a few; see Scott 1969: 21ff. and Monbeck 1973), are very real expectations that persons have for their own vision loss and future life-course.

Most people who go through adventitious vision loss share the mistaken belief of the world at large that blindness is deserving of pity. One person succinctly observed that 'I felt like it [blindness] was a big, big handicap. I felt that they probably had great big problems, you know? And I felt sorry for them.' Very often their feelings toward blindness were developed in their interaction with people they had known before the advent of their own visual difficulties. One individual spoke of a person that she had seen around her home town over the years.

> Before I had the problem with my own eyes I'd see a blind person and say 'Oh, a blind person,' you know? That was the worst thing that could happen. It was so terrible before when I'd think of it. I'd think of complete darkness, pitch black. I'd think of it at its worst, you know?

Another spoke of her many years of giving contributions to blindness agencies and the feelings conjured up in her mind.

> We always used to get the booklets, you know? And I'd always send money for the Association for the Blind. I always thought, well, you know, like sometimes you hear 'I'd rather be dead than blind.' Well, that's what I thought. I thought I would be unable to cope with it.

Another person told of watching a young person with blindness pass his home. Each day as the person would pass the house, he would note to himself,

> He'd just go by on his way to the store. He'd tap his cane around the curb and if somebody would talk to him he'd say 'Hi.' He's young, you know? Not very old. You feel sorry when you see people walking with a cane like that.

Other people had closer personal contact with blindness, yet pity remained their predominant response and their fear of their own blindness seemed magnified. One individual recalled her years of taking care of her father.

> My dad was blind the last two or three years before he died. I would have to pour his milk, his juice, pour his tea. You don't know the messes he'd make in the daytime. He'd think he'd have the glass in his hand and he would just tip it, you know? And we'd have to cut the food on his plate like that and

everything. I couldn't have ever believed that I would get that way too.

Rather than easing the anticipation of their own sensory decline, such direct, personal experience of, and exposure to, blindness seemed most often to confirm their worst fears about the problems vision loss would bring.

In many cases, the astonishment with which they viewed the mundane accomplishments of persons with blindness (accomplishments they would have taken for granted of a person with sight) betrayed the low expectations they actually held.

I had a lot of blind customers who would come into my store. I used to appreciate them because I could see there were a lot of things that they could do for themselves. I knew a blind person, I won't mention his name, who would come into my shop. He'd walk three-quarters of a mile. He'd take a chair by himself and sit down. He'd get up when he was ready to leave, feel the door knob and open the door by himself. I admired him for that. I used to think a lot of him. I said 'A person that's blind can really help himself. That's wonderful.'

These accomplishments, however, seemed to pale in their significance once the person realized that these would be the same criteria by which she/he would now be judged.

Almost as if to postpone these judgements, it was quite common for people to develop what Shontz calls 'defensive avoidance techniques' (1975: 147). This is to say that many became well practiced at 'as if' behavior. They seemed to believe that the pain and the fear of new vision loss could be avoided by simply trying to act 'as if' it didn't exist. As one person reported,

Of course, there are some days when it is not too good. I just don't feel like I can do anything. So I just say 'Well, it's one of those days.' I lock the door and I take off. I go down the street or I go walking. See people that I know. Go on a coffee break. Anything, you know, so long as I get out of the house. And I just don't talk about my sight at all. I will talk about anything else, you know? Like now, it is almost Christmas so we will talk about Christmas shopping, how much we have done. Anything you know? I keep away from the subject.

People acknowledge that such defensive avoidance techniques retard their efforts to come to terms with their new lives. The overriding purpose-at-hand, however, tends to lie with avoiding the all-too-apparent impact of their vision loss on their day-to-day lives. This is often accomplished by focusing on those projects and tasks which remain within the range of activities as yet unaffected by their visual impairment.

As Shontz further notes, avoidance techniques are related to, but conceptually separable from, denial of the impairment. According to Dover (1959), her studies of newly visually-impaired persons seem to indicate a series of denial mechanisms which complement these avoidance techniques. Dover (1959: 336) notes, 'denial is frequently expressed through assertions that hope cannot be abandoned, that new medical discoveries are being made all the time and that this condition may be subject to change by some magical means and so on.' As suggested earlier, often the person with no medical or surgical recourse will seek out unorthodox remedies in an effort to provide themselves with some hope beyond what is offered by current medical technology. Others continue to maintain that advances could still be made which would restore their visual functioning. The following response was common:

> I say the worst thing in the world is to lose your eyesight. But my hope is that someday they can find, you know, different ways to avoid the problem entirely. So people like me can help their sight, you know? It is a lot to ask and I know they will have to do a lot of work on it before it happens. Sometimes I imagine that I will never get the chance to have it but I am hoping.

These denial mechanisms serve as a buffer to the otherwise oppressive awareness that their life has been so severely disrupted.

Bodily discontinuity and identity

It has been suggested that it is the body which accompanies people throughout their involvement in the world, provides them with a sense of both space and time, and mediates their actions in and upon their environment. Inasmuch as people are coextensive with their bodies, their experience of their situation, continuity, and character – their identity – is inextricably bound with their experience of their biological organism. This is to say that one must necessarily account for people's bodily experience as it acts upon and is, in turn, interpreted by people's subjective experience of themselves.

As advancing age often carries with it a series of disruptions to people's organismic experience, it affords a particularly unique opportunity to see the interplay of body and consciousness in flux. The progression of vision loss, the changing relationship that people have with the physical world that surrounds them, changes in their sense of time and space, altered recipes, and the like, all call into question the world taken for granted and pose for the individual an indisputably 'problematic' situation.

As Simone de Beauvoir has observed, 'deterioration is inevitable: no man escapes it' (1972: 302). Yet biological decline can be fast or slow, more nearly partial or entire, and can vary in the intensity with which it affects an individual's life. The loss of sight is usually a slow but steady process which ultimately creates a sort of crisis situation which does, indeed, intensely affect the person's hold on the world in which she/he had always considered her/himself to be an integral part.

The preceding discussion has tried to offer evidence that new vision loss is, by no means, just one characteristic among others. It curtails people's abilities to realize even the most mundane of their intentions such as the ability to consume food. It makes the once-familiar surroundings of their home seem a hostile and unknowable environment. It makes such activities as reading, writing, shopping, driving, and even walking short distances, seem like insurmountable challenges. It constantly reminds people of just how essential visual cues can be to making decisions about which action is appropriate to a given situation, and confronts them with their own susceptibility to errors in judgement. In short, the loss of this crucial sensory skill makes the individual acutely aware of the perhaps seemingly-innocuous statement 'the body determines which projects are within reach.'

To a great extent, then, new vision loss accompanying the aging process calls into question the appropriateness of a large number of the personal recipes which people once used almost unthinkingly to manipulate their physical space. They are no longer confident that 'I-can-do-it-again' and as such each situation becomes potentially originary, requiring a whole series of new and often improvised recipes. In a world largely ordered by visual cues and signals, people's attempts to reintegrate their lives into the unproblematic are continually frustrated.

People's very sense of the space and the time are brought into relief by new vision loss. Because objects become both hostile and unknowable, people may become disoriented, which is to say that the physical reality which surrounds them loses its coherency and it is not readily understandable to them. The terms they once used while sighted to order their world may now be inappropriate. In affirmation of what phenomenologists insist is the intentional nature of lived experience, new vision loss demonstrates the full impact of the dictum: people exist for objects and objects exist for people. People are given new hardware such as the cane with which they are supposed to relearn how to manipulate space, but they are never able to replace the visual background which they once took for granted and they remain constantly aware of its absence. Persons with visual impairments become increasingly present oriented. While they may treasure their recollections of perceptions now lost, they cannot allow themselves the luxury of dwelling upon the past because of the challenges to their present, and they cannot plan ahead because of the uncertainties of the future. In sum, new vision loss affects people's ability to act upon both time and space. It constricts their so-called life/space extensity.

While it would be inaccurate to speak of established stages that a person goes through in losing her/his eyesight, there are a number of common initial reactions which are shared by most people who experience vision loss. To greater and lesser extents, and in varying order of experience, most go through some disbelief, anger, shock, hope, puzzlement, and panic. They express realistic anxieties about what their future will hold and these are often compounded by their preconceptions of what vision loss threatens. As has been shown, they often attempt to avoid and/or deny the organismic decline which has become so obvious to them. De Beauvoir insists that 'in the first place, we have to live in [old age], experience it, in our bodies' (1972: 301). For aging persons with new vision loss, this experience of the body forces them to confront the limitations which are imposed by a bodily vehicle that no longer carries them through day-to-day experience in the ways they had become accustomed through the years. Their experiences of their bodies therefore challenge their sense of personal continuity throughout time and place, their grasp of their situation in the world, and their very notion of their personal character. Many projects are now cut off from them, just as is the visual background in which their expression had traditionally taken place. Persons with new vision loss, then, must come to grips in an exaggerated way with what all older persons must eventually face: 'the old man's tragedy is that often he is no longer capable of what he desires' (de Beauvoir 1972: 315).

The fallibility of the body has, of course, profound impact on a person's identity. Butler and Lewis have noted that

> older people's sense of pride in their own body's reliability is
> shaken when they experience their greater susceptibility to

communicable diseases, air pollution, dampness, cold weather and exertion. Moreover, aging and disease threaten people's sense of who they are – their identities – as their bodies change in front of their eyes. (1977: 39)

In a similar fashion, but even more so, sensory decline not only shakes a person's pride in her/his body's reliability, but it threatens her/his sense of identity as it is lived – that is, as it is conceived and fulfilled in a world. It is, in many ways, no longer the same world, precisely because her/his relationship to its objects has been so dramatically altered. It is the dramatic nature of these changes in their world, or more accurately in the world as it is available to them, which prompts the reactions surveyed thus far.

The interruptions in recipes by which they made the world have meaning, the curtailment of their activities once taken for granted, their equivocal hold on space and the time, all make it impossible for people to accept their lives in 'self evident and compelling facticity' – the way in which ordinary people experience their lives (Berger and Luckmann 1966). The world once available is no longer simply there. In a word, people experience their new vision loss as discontinuous with the life they once knew and which they simply accepted as 'real.' Their faith in their ability to realize intentions upon the world having been shaken by their newly-discovered organismic fallibility, their bodies no longer supplying them with the sensory information upon which they had relied so heavily, and their uncertain future, force persons also to question the whole sense in which they once considered themselves to be 'alive.' Lastly, the unknowable and hostile character of the objects around them persuade people to question their once-assumed experiential unity with the world around them, the sense in which they once considered themselves as 'whole.' Vision loss accompanying the aging process therefore challenges people's experience of their own being as real, alive, and whole, or, in R.D. Laing's (1960) words, it challenges a person's 'ontological security.' As such it raises questions for people about their own genuineness, inner consistency, substantiality, and worth. It challenges their identity. How these challenges are resolved (if they are) can only be understood in terms of the social context within which vision loss occurs and the individual's ultimate capacity to restore a sense of ontological security to her/his life in spite of these discontinuities in their relationship between her/his conscious expression in the world and her/his bodily experience.

Moreover, this dramatic change in the world creates the very possibility that persons may see themselves as 'abnormal.' As

Berger and Luckmann note, 'abnormality becomes a biographical possibility if a certain competition exists between reality definitions, raising the possibility of choosing between them' (1966: 168). Reality definitions, like identity itself, evolve in-the-world, which is to say in the relationship that exists between consciousness and physical and social worlds. With the disruption of a person's visual capacity to receive and interpret the world around her/him, one's normal sighted sense of self is counterposed by a competing view of subjective reality as abnormal. As will be seen, the ultimate outcome of this struggle can only be understood within a social context yet to be discussed, but it becomes a possibility by virtue of the discontinuities of one's old sighted versus one's new visually-impaired experience of the world.

Chapter three
Changing relationships with others

Visually-impaired persons do not come to terms with their biological and sensory decline in a social vacuum. On the contrary, people's reactions to, and even the nature of, their experiences of vision loss are, in large part, tempered by the social environment in which they find themselves. As such, the social environment as well as the physical environment already discussed are important components in what is the dialectical interplay of identity. In fact, consistent with the way in which phenomenologists have used the hyphen (being-in-the-world, etc.), the phrase 'identity-in-the-world' might be more appropriate terminology (see Ainlay and Redfoot 1982 for a more detailed discussion of this concept). This is intended to suggest the interconnectedness of people's own interpretations of continuity, situation, and character – their identity (as broadly defined by Goffman 1963) – with the world that surrounds them. Just as a person's understanding of her/himself is undeniably linked to her/his body, so too is the experience of the social world critical to self estimations. In Peter Berger's terms 'the individual realizes himself in society – that is, he recognizes his identity in socially defined terms and these definitions become reality as he lives in society' (1970: 375). The social world, therefore, serves both to maintain and confirm the subjective reality termed identity. This, of course, raises the possibility that the social world can also fail to maintain or may disconfirm a particular subjective reality (which is quite clear in the case of conversion, see Berger and Luckmann's discussion of this process, 1966: 157ff.).

Along with the organismic access to the physical world around them, it is people's social involvements which demand that identity always be conceived of as 'in-the-world' and not merely an ethereal entity. The questions which this chapter seeks to address are therefore all related to broad issues surrounding the inter-play of people with their social environment and the mechanisms of the latter for reality maintenance/modification and reality confirmation/disconfirmation.

Vision loss and its impact on communication

Communication makes social life itself possible. It is through communication that people make their intentions known, pass on information to novices and succeeding generations and even establish 'we' vs 'they.' It is particularly important to people's self appraisals of their situation, continuity, and character. This importance of communication has been most often acknowledged in discussions of language. Berger and Luckmann, for example, insist that 'language . . . typifies experiences allowing me to subsume them under broad categories in terms of which they have meaning not only to myself but also to my fellowmen' (1966: 39). As such, language is one of the chief instruments by which people make sense of their worlds. With specific regard to identity, language provides people with the terms by which self appraisals can be generated and maintained, as well as the mechanism whereby the appraisals of others are conveyed. Yet spoken language is only one part of the communicative process. Para-linguistic expression is important as well, as has been demonstrated by various writers; Birdwhistell (1970 and 1973), through his 'kinesics' (the science of body behavioral communication), and others working in the area of 'nonverbal' communication, have successfully argued the importance of posture, distance, eye contact, and other factors in interactive encounters and in signaling one's estimations of others.

Vision is very important to the process of communication and can become an indicator of a person's character. Robert Scott argues that

> Vision plays an enormously important role in personal communication. When we speak to someone, it is customary for us to maintain eye contact. This is learned from the earliest age, so that by about the time a child begins school, this very important lesson has been learned. To turn away or focus on a distant object when addressing another person can be attributed to rudeness, shyness, or guilt. Frequently the lack of visual contact is one of the factors responsible for the statement, 'We simply could not communicate.' Eye contact signifies honesty, directness, attentiveness, respect and a variety of other virtues that are the important ingredients of successful human communication. (1969: 30)

Similar arguments have been made by Simmel (1970), Kendon (1973), and Argyle and Dean (1973). The disruption of sight, then, poses a serious threat to the interaction through which communication with others occurs, and may raise questions about the very character of the person who experiences vision loss.

The loss of sight most dramatically affects the person's ability to manipulate the 'mechanics' of communication successfully (Scott 1969: 32). The full meaning of Scott's discussion of the importance of vision loss was readily apparent to those who, for example, reported

> You have some family problems on account of your vision problem. You know, sometimes they thought that I didn't want to talk to them. But I didn't know they were there. Somebody would be sitting there but I wouldn't recognize them except if they talked or something like that. Some of them thought that I didn't want to have anything to do with them so I had a few problems like that.

Or again

> I go out and I don't know people. This is one of the things that bothers me. Like I could meet you out there and I wouldn't know who you were. So I keep telling people, 'it's not that I'm snubbing you.' Sometimes people feel that you are turning them off or ignoring them or something. But it's not that, it's just because I don't, I can't see them.

Quite often this problem is exacerbated by people's reluctance to admit to others that they can no longer see well enough to communicate as they once did.

> At first I wouldn't tell people that my eyes were that bad. I just felt maybe they would get better and I wouldn't have to tell them, I guess. You know? I says, 'I'll wait', and I wouldn't tell them. But then you meet people and they'll say, 'Gee, I saw you and you didn't look at me.' Well, I didn't see them, you know? After a while it made me nervous. I would go downtown and would kind of look around and I couldn't spot them. That bothered me. I couldn't see the people I knew so then I finally had to come out and tell them, 'If you see me, touch me as you go by or say, hi, so I can talk with you.'

A number of people reported going to great lengths to hide their vision loss by working around circumstances which would expose their visual incompetence. The following example of eating in a restaurant is representative of these efforts.

> Sometimes you can cover it [vision loss] up. I'd kind of fake it, you know? Like I'd go into a restaurant. Well I couldn't read the menu so I'd ask the waitress, 'What's the special of the day?' I can still fake it pretty good. Some of them still don't know that I can't read the menu.

The ruse is surprisingly easy for many to pull off, at least for a while. Unlike persons blind throughout their lives or accidentally blinded (described by Scott 1969: 31), whose eyes may be disconcerting to the sighted observer, most persons in this study (and this is typical of most elderly persons who are blind) showed little visible evidence of their visual disorder. This is often compounded by their continued wearing of eye glasses which, in actual fact, no longer aid their vision but which they feel have some cosmetic appeal (and may play a part in what Goffman [1963] terms 'covering strategies'). Only the slight tilt of the head away from the speaker or slight discoloration of the eye evidence the telltale signs of the severity of their loss. Their impairment is not always 'visible.' Social scientists have failed to appreciate this fact and, as such, have often miscategorized the blind or addressed the experience of only a few. Goffman, in his landmark book *Stigma* (1963: 48), speaks of the blind as being 'readily visible' and argues that it is therefore very difficult for them to 'pass' (that is, to cover-up 'stigma symbols' so that other people will not identify them as belonging to a stigmatized group). While this analysis may work for the relatively small number of blind and visually-impaired persons who manifest obvious external signs of their vision loss, it obscures the experience of most older persons (again, the bulk of the total population that is blind and visually impaired).

Newly visually-impaired persons may seek to pass or hide their vision loss with good reason. Many people reported that their visual impairment led to a certain reluctance on the part of their sighted friends to include them in conversations as they did before its onset.

> Some people are uncomfortable around me. Especially some who see me with a cane don't like it. Sometimes people that you know won't come and talk with you. You know? You sometimes wonder what's going on but I think that it's just they don't know what to do. They don't feel at ease with you. They are afraid that they are gonna do the wrong thing or say the wrong thing.

Goffman (1957, 1963) has discussed at great length the uneasiness of 'normals' in interaction with stigmatized individuals. As Stafford and Scott (1986) note, their uneasiness may bespeak fear, vengeance, or even the desire to control the other socially. Regardless of reason, their uneasiness often leads people with sight to exclude visually-impaired persons from full participation in conversations. Often the visually-impaired individual finds her/himself on the periphery of the dialogue.

> What really gets me – it's happened since I've lost my sight – is that I'll be with somebody else and we'll meet somebody and we start talking and all of a sudden they are talking and I am kind of left out on the side, you know? They'll talk and there you are on the side, you know? They'll talk and there you are on the side and you feel like 'what am I doing here?' Well, I have to butt in to get in on it.

As Goffman says, the individual becomes a 'non-person' and is treated like he/she isn't there at all (1963: 18). At other times people mistakenly believe they are being excluded because they fail to pick out the interactive cues which signal their inclusion in the conversation.

> Somebody may be speaking to me and I don't know that he's looking at me. You know normally we look at each other when we talk. Say I'm talking to you and I'll say, 'Are you going anywhere tonight?' If you see me looking at you, you know I'm talking to you. Well, I won't know that. I won't know if he's addressing me or not.

Both the feeling of being excluded and this inability to pick up on visual cues discourage the person and create strains in the communication process itself. People are often, therefore, reluctant to seek out interaction with those around them.

A distressing consequence of new vision loss may therefore be the reduced opportunity to articulate one's view of self to others. The usual process by which others express their views of the situation and of the person's very character may be curtailed. At a time when people are struggling to achieve some sense of personal continuity between their previously-sighted life and their new life with a visual impairment, this cutoff from day-to-day conversation leaves them without a most important vehicle for maintaining subjective reality. In a very real sense it may signal to individuals that they no longer share a common world with their sighted associates. Ultimately, this makes the person vulnerable to alternative and sometimes competing social worlds. In the case of people who are visually impaired, they become drawn to the world of persons of like circumstance and the so-called 'blindness system.'

The reaction of others to vision loss

While we must guard against being overly deterministic, there is no doubt that the reactions of those around us have an enormous impact upon the formation of our personal agenda, our attitudes toward the world, and indeed our sense of self. It is clear that a person's experience of visual and hence organismic decline always occurs within the context of a social environment. This environment is composed not only of general day-to-day contacts with other people but is, in large part, influenced by, and at times directed from, the vantage of those 'significant others' whose attitudes toward the individual become a crucial ingredient in the creation and maintenance of her/his subjective reality. In the words of Berger and Luckmann,

> To retain confidence that he is indeed who he thinks he is, the individual requires not only the implicit confirmation of his identity that even casual everyday contacts will supply, but the explicit and emotionally charged confirmation that his significant others bestow on him. (1966: 150)

For newly visually-impaired persons, the realization of their organismic limitations flows not only from the difficulties they experience in relearning their relation with the object world but also from the reactions to their loss that others, both significant and less significant, exhibit to them.

Perhaps most important to aging individuals are the reactions of their immediate family – spouse (if that person survives), children, as well as other family members. Together these people share the loss of vision and the recognition of the changes implied. As Carlos Neu has observed, 'relatives, especially those who live close to the blind person, suffer the loss just as seriously and that affects their lives profoundly' (1975: 2,161). They are, as Goffman (1963) terms them, the 'wise.' Their own personal relation to the object world is, of course, unchanged. Yet, because of their closeness to the visually-impaired person, they have a sort of surrogate experience of the resulting frustrations, fears, disbelief, and anger. In fact, in the words of one individual, it is sometimes apparent that 'it bothers them a lot more than it bothers me.' Another person echoed this sentiment and reported that his son, for example, refused to come to terms with his loss of vision.

It took my boy a long time to get adjusted, you know, to the fact that I was blind. When we'd go somewhere it was next to impossible for him to take me by the arm, to lead me. It took him a long time to get adjusted and to realize that it was so and a fact of life. He's a good boy but he had problems. We have always been very close and I really think that he just felt, 'It can't happen to my father.' 'It shouldn't happen to him.' I don't really know why – that's just my personal thought.

Becoming 'wise' is not something that occurs immediately. Most people reported that family members experienced this initial disbelief in their physical fallibility. For some this reaction of their family added to the 'hurt' of the physical loss. One individual, speaking of his wife's initial disbelief, suggested that, while troubled by her reaction, he understood her feelings.

Well, at first I was a little bit hurt but then I understood what she was going through. I don't know that if my wife became blind tomorrow that I wouldn't act the same way. It would be hard for me to realize that she had become blind.

Thus, the person's sense of disbelief in her/his own physical fallibility is often shared with and confirmed by family members.

Family members share in a number of other reactions to vision loss as well. Some people reported that spouse and/or children sometimes exhibited an intense anger at the vision loss only rivaled by the individual's own ire. Others suggested that their own embarrassment was accompanied by what they perceived to be the uneasiness of family when accompanying them in a public setting. Goffman (1963) suggests that it is common for family members of a person with some stigmatized condition to have a sort of 'courtesy stigma' (a sort of stigma by association) and this may well contribute to the sense of embarrassment. Most commonly, however, people reported that, just as they had themselves often tried to avoid their vision loss by keeping busy or talking about other things, their family systematically seemed to avoid the subject whenever possible. As one person noted of her husband's reaction,

He always kind of avoided the subject. When I would go downtown to see the ophthalmologist, why he'd go along with me but he never would talk about it. It was just one of those things, you know, that he never said too much about.

Several people noted that, when talking over the phone with children who no longer lived in the area, there was a conspicuous avoidance of the subject of their vision loss. People who are visually impaired seldom initiate the topic, not wanting to dwell on their problems or indulge themselves in what might be interpreted as self pity.

This avoidance of the subject of vision loss often leads to avoidance of the person experiencing it as well. One of the inter-active problems which nearly every person mentioned revolved around the apparent efforts of friends to avoid contact with the individual after the onset of visual impairment. As Monbeck has noted, one of the most common reactions to blindness throughout history has been that of derision and avoidance (1973: 54) and, as Siller *et al.* (1967: 61–2) empirically confirm, that avoidance is one of the most common of responses. The following experience is typical.

> You will go to a reception somewhere – you know a wedding or a funeral or something like that – and there are always a lot of people there you have not seen for a long time and you would like to see. Well, you happen to think about them or ask someone about them and they will say, 'Oh, he was here and he just left a few minutes ago.' They won't come to you. They won't come to let you know they are there. I guess they feel bashful.

Another person suggests that this happens nearly all the time and hints at her personal reaction to the realization that she is being avoided.

> Before, when I had my eyesight, people would always say, hello, and talk to me. Now that they know I can't see, they don't always. It's one thing I've noticed. They will just go by you. They figure that just because you can't see, your sight is bad, that they can just walk by. They say, 'Well, she can't see me anyway.' If I'm with somebody they will say, 'Well, there is so and so going by.' You expect them to say, hi, or do something so you will know it is them. So you can talk to them, you know? Well, that hurts and it happens a lot.

While it is possible to posit a variety of unconscious psychological motivations to this avoidance (i.e. fear, 'emotional syllogism,' belief in the evil-like nature of the blind, etc.; see Monbeck 1973: 108) it seems more plausible that most people's avoidance of visually-impaired friends is rooted in their anxiety about the anticipated interaction which is made uncertain by the presumed interactive incompetence of their visually-impaired associate. This has been experimentally demonstrated by Kleck *et al.* (1966) and is consistent with the observations of Goffman (1957) and Fred

Davis (1964) as well. Their concern with the awkwardness of the interaction and their belief that the visually-impaired person will be unable to 'hold her/his own' in a face-to-face encounter are sufficient reasons for the sighted person to avoid interaction with their now visually-impaired friends (without seeking underlying unconscious motivations). Thus visually-impaired persons frequently reported that their vision loss prompted either abbreviated or total cutoffs of interaction with long-term friends and acquaintances.

Interestingly, in a number of cases the reverse situation was reported. For those who still had remaining sight and showed no visible signs of their vision loss, often they were frustrated by people's expectations for their full participation in the world of others. One individual, for example, insisted that several of his close friends refused to believe that his sight was actually worsening and chose, rather, to suggest he was seeking additional tax advantages. Another person told of his own brother's suspicion of his motives. On several different occasions he reported that his brother would actually 'test' him. For example,

> This brother of mine is always saying, 'What the hell do you use a cane for? You're not blind.' And one time he stood in front of me in a row in my garden for ten minutes until I finally ran into him. He laughed like heck. He said, 'You're not blind.'

People spoke of their frustrations: on the one hand at being unable to do the things they once took for granted; and on the other at people's insistence that they were in some way 'faking' their impairment. This, of course, happened in relatively few cases, yet it seems that it is a potential complication to the onset of vision loss which may occur for those who do not have a 'visible' impairment.

Common to family, friends, and even casual contacts in daily life is the tendency to overcompensate for the person's vision loss. Visually-impaired persons are greatly aware of people's efforts to avoid such words as 'see.' One person, for example, reported his amusement at people who nearly choke on the phrase 'I'll see you later.' They exhibit their uneasiness with visual impairment in other ways as well.

> Some people over-react, they try to over help me. They grab me by the arm or underneath the arm and they'll push me here or pull me there. Somebody will come up to shake my hand and they'll flip my hand way up in the air. I guess they're embarrassed that I don't see. I know they embarrass me more than a little bit. They push it too far, you know?

There is also a tendency for others to attribute a host of disabilities to the visually-impaired person which are totally irrelevant to the loss of vision. Persons who are blind frequently report, for instance, that sighted people talk loudly with them as if to assume that their vision loss has affected their hearing. One individual in this study suggested that this imputation of sensory incompetence may extend to smell as well. She recalled,

> We had just got some new furniture and the cushion in the chair – well it smelled musty. So I called the furniture store and told them. Well they didn't believe me. So I told my husband when he got home, 'Just because I can't see they think I can't smell, either.' You know it's just like your hearing. When people talk with you they holler because they think you can't hear, either. I guess it's a natural reaction.

Sometimes this imputation of additional sensory decline will lead to further exclusion from the interactive process itself. Most people were able to recall instances when a question about them was addressed to their spouse or someone else who accompanied them. For example, the following restaurant scene was common:

> When you're in a restaurant why they will ask your husband if you want sugar or cream in your tea instead of asking you. I guess they think you can't answer for yourself if you can't see.

Imputations of character occur all the time in everyday interaction. It is that part of a person which Goffman calls one's 'virtual social identity.' In other words, people commonly 'make certain assumptions about what the individual before us ought to be' (1963: 2). People act toward one another as if people possessed certain characteristics 'in effect.' In the case of new vision loss, however, these imputations of character often turn toward the expectation of further incompetencies and can lead to additional patterns of avoidance or over-compensation.

As one listens to the newly visually-impaired person recount her/his life since the onset of vision difficulties, it becomes readily apparent that the frustrations, fears, and uneasiness she/he has with regard to the body's physical fallibility is compounded by the social environment in which she/he finds her/himself embedded. Indeed, the family and friends of the visually-impaired person seem to share in the anger, the frustrations, and disbelief that she/he has come to know. The similarities in their common response to vision loss are, of course, partly rooted in their shared preconceptions of what vision loss implies and their shared anticipations of the uncertainty of the future life course. As people begin to relearn the recipes by which they will confront and interpret their new, visually-impaired lives, these reactions of significant others and the 'chorus' of casual contacts tend to confirm their own perceptions of biological demise. In this way 'self and society are inextricably interwoven entities' (Berger 1970: 375). The person's own estimation of her/his new situation is compounded by and inseparable from the estimation of others. Together they reshape the very relationships of the visually-impaired person to those around her/him, the physical world, and even her/his biological organism, the body itself. For the most part, as will be seen in the following discussion, in defining a new relationship with the world the visually-impaired person must incorporate the limitations imposed by the actual vision loss as well as the limitations which are socially imposed.

Socially imposed limitations to activity

In Chapter 2 a number of the obstacles imposed upon the activities of the visually-impaired person by virtue of the loss of sight were discussed. The curtailment of activities, just as any other dimension of the experience of new vision loss, occurs within a social context. It is this same context, the social environment, which often confirms the person's inability to carry on as usual and which in many cases exaggerates the limitations which have been physically imposed.

In part, because they impute a whole series of delimited expectations upon the newly visually-impaired person (as part of their virtual identity) and in part because they seek to create a sort of protective capsule within which he/she can safely reside, family and friends often respond to a person's new vision loss in an overly-protective fashion. As Goffman (1963: 332) has noted, they create this 'protective capsule' to prevent belittling treatments by the outside world from affecting the visually-impaired person (and correspondingly themselves). Beyond this, in the case of new vision loss, it also seems that they create this protective capsule in an effort to insulate their loved one from what they perceive to be physical dangers of the outside world and in the hopes that they can minimize some of the frustrations which the person feels because they can no longer easily complete all the tasks they once readily accomplished.

Some of the concern for the person's well-being is prompted by the warnings of the medical community. For example, common to those whose vision loss was due to a retinal detachment was the belief that too much activity would risk additional if not total loss of sight. As one person with a retinal detachment reported,

> I was afraid to do something that might make me get totally blind sooner, you know? Like old Dr Porter in town here, he told me that there were a lot of things I shouldn't do like lifting anything. So I didn't. It wasn't until years later that I went to Boston where I guess the doctors are more knowledgeable, and they said, unless I really strained, if you're going to get a detachment you are going to get it. They said you would have to fall flat on your face or something would have to hit you on the back of your head. But that could happen no matter what you did.

Whether prompted by a doctor's warning or simply flowing from the commonsensical presumption of the person's new vulnerability, the families of the newly visually-impaired persons universally sought to protect them from physical injury. The following description of family reaction was typical.

> My family was overprotective. I had to fight them when I was ready to resume my life as it was before. It is only just lately that I can get out of their sight to go down the street. . . . And the moment I tried to do something, they'd come and do it for me, you know? They would never ask me to do anything. They would do it themselves.

This overprotectiveness extends from the privacy of the home to the public environment as well. People reported that, as they would go out into their respective communities, people were always anticipating that they would in some way hurt themselves. Again the following example is representative.

> The other day I went to city hall to see the city clerk about some business. I am used to the city hall and have been there many times. But every time I go there the city clerk is so protective. She's afraid that I'll fall down the stairs and all that. They try to help you a lot more than they should, you know? Sometimes they'll grab you by the hand or something like that. You can see that they are nervous about it.

This sense of others' nervousness and constant guarding against the possibility that the individual may injure her/himself often puts the visually-impaired person on edge. There is little doubt that it confirms and magnifies the tentativeness with which they naturally begin to approach the world around them. As Jervis (1964) has noted, there is ample evidence that this protective attitude of family members curtails interaction with their social environment.

The overprotectiveness of those around the visually-impaired person, especially family members, often encourages a sort of social dependency. This fact has been observed in much of the literature on aging. Clausen, for example, has observed,

> In infancy the individual's only power is that which he exercises by virtue of the love his parents have for him; his dependency is absolute. Through the childhood years his dependency lessens and changes in nature, and his power to influence others increases. In adulthood, power is closely linked to occupational role, except as power over one's children is concerned; one is supposed to be self-dependent. For the infirm adult or one who loses his source of livelihood, dependency again becomes a major problem. (in Riley *et al.* 1972: 511)

As Kubler-Ross has noted, this sort of dependency is not some sort of psychological maladaption but is rather 'no less than a realistic response to the social situation in which they are placed' (1975: 18).

For the visually-impaired older person, this dependency is encouraged by the family's and friends' attempts to do things for the individual and, correspondingly, to take away her/his very power to act upon the world around her/him. A typical illustration was offered by one person regarding her friends' actions.

> Some of them they'll go overboard in trying to help you and it makes you feel like you can't do it. I mean of course you've lost your eyesight but it makes you feel that you've lost something so important like your eyesight and so you can't do it. They do it out of kindness but they shouldn't do it. Like pouring coffee, I'll have friends in and they'll be so afraid that I would burn myself, you know? And they would say, 'Why don't you let me pour the coffee?' I wanted to do things for myself but like I say friends would go a little overboard and make you feel like you can't handle it.

For visually-impaired persons, many of the day-to-day activities which they seek to accomplish do indeed require the cooperation and aid of sighted others. As Scott observes, this 'charitable' behavior can have demoralizing and humiliating effects (1969: 37). The strain of the new-found dependency upon the charity of others can be very difficult for the newly visually-impaired person to accommodate.

You see somebody with poor eyesight, you just want to help them. You know, you can do things better and faster, you know? I felt that way before too. I'd see somebody with poor eyes and they were having a hard time so I thought I wanted to do things for them, you know? I've found that it takes a long time before you can accept help though. Because you feel like you want to do it. But you sometimes have to learn that you do have to ask for help. You have to let people help you.

Visually-impaired persons eventually relearn to do many things for themselves. But contrary to the rehabilitation ideology that suggests one can become entirely self-sufficient, most newly visually-impaired persons come to the realization that a certain dependency upon the cooperation of the sighted world is necessary for them to live in a world with many visual cues. As Van Weelden observes, this awareness of their dependency on others further contributes to visually-impaired persons' sense of ambivalence toward their bodies (1967: 57). It socially confirms not only the difficulty of maintaining the façade of visual competence but constantly reminds them of the limitations their vision loss places upon their very freedom to create a world ongoingly, a 'freedom' to which most others are continually 'condemned' (see Sartre 1953).

Changing social network

One of the most certain characteristics of aging is the inevitable changes it imposes upon a person's circle of family and close friends, her/his social network. As Burgess accurately noted, 'family and friends are important at all ages, but are subject to their greatest strain and breaking-up in old age' (1950: 155). There are, of course, many reasons why the social network of the elderly visually-impaired person begins to dissolve. Many of these reasons do not actually stem from the loss of vision but rather are related to changes that occur characteristically in any aging cohort. In the light of their relatively closer proximity to death, for example, it is not surprising that the older visually-impaired person is confronted with widowhood or the passing of friends and other relatives. Almost every individual, in discussing relations with others, lamented the deaths of spouses, children, siblings, and friends who had once been so important a part of life. In the words of one 86 year old,

I'll bet you I knew over 95 per cent of all the people in this town. 'Cause my work kept me in the streets a lot, you know –

the plumbing, the repairing and everything. Why I knew everyone from the hooker on the street to the doctors and the lawyers to the ministers and the priests. I knew them all. We had a wonderful life but the way it is now I don't see that it will get any better. Everyone of my really good friends is dead now. I haven't got any of my old friends. My father and mother is over there in the cemetery. My brother too. He got his in the First World War. My wife is over there. And, of course, there's room for me.

These losses have their impact not only on the person's pool of potential interactions but often leave the person without the support (material and emotional) which might make the loss of vision seem less isolating and perhaps less disruptive. With their deaths, however, vision loss becomes one more loss among others.

Well, my life has changed quite a bit. See I started my problem with my eyes and then my husband died. So then I had to sell my house and move into an apartment downtown. And those were things I hadn't planned on. I always thought my husband would be with me for the rest of my life. I guess you never think about him actually dying. He had a heart attack. It was fast. When he died, I already knew I was going to lose my eyesight. I've always felt that if he was with me it would be easier to take. I'd be with him and I could share things, you know? Tell him things. If I had had my husband maybe I could have gone on as before.

As Rose has observed, 'when one of an older couple dies, the remaining person is cut off from his major social contact' (1961: 463).

The same is, of course, true of the death of other family members and of close friends, together with whom the person once shared a social world and upon whom their sense of subjective reality also relied. As de Beauvoir notes, 'The death of a friend, of one who was close to us, not only deprives us of a presence but of a whole of that part of our lives that was committed to them' (1972: 366). Further, death is only one of an array of other means by which the aging person's social network may begin to break up. Retirement to another state, institutional-ization in nursing facilities and the like, chronic illness, all tend either to minimize or dissolve interaction among significant others. The death of family and friends as well as these other factors make the social networks, within which people traditionally maintained and confirmed their sense of self, at best equivocal.

There are a variety of factors which are directly related to vision loss which contribute toward the breakdown of one's social network as well. Most commonly, visually-impaired persons find that the tendency of old friends to avoid the presumed awkwardness of interaction (as discussed earlier) often leads to a total breakdown in their old patterns of association. People commonly reported that they were almost mystified as to why they were no longer invited to the homes of friends whom they had known for years. Others felt they knew all too well why old friends didn't stop by or invite them out any more.

> I think that one of the worst parts of my adjustment [to vision loss] was the people. I didn't feel like they had the same feeling towards me after I lost my eyesight. I guess they figured me for a blind person. It seemed as though things were different. A lot of my old friends didn't want to bother with me or didn't know how to cope or whatever it was. I don't know. I had some personal friends and they'd see me around the yard and they'd stop to talk with me. Once. I'd never see them again. They'd say, 'I'll be back and talk with you' or 'We'll go somewhere.' But they never did. It didn't seem to me that there was any reason for a cutoff. I don't know how they saw a cause for a cutoff. That hurts – naturally.

This breakdown of interaction between old friends is not always a one-sided affair. Several people reported that they had stopped asking friends over after they began to lose their vision. In large, they curtailed their contacts with old friends because they felt uneasy about their visual difficulties and worried that they would do something embarrassing. Several single or widowed persons suggested that since they could no longer see to clean their house they would never have the courage to ask old friends over to their home.

For many of the people this breakdown of their old relationships left them without an active social life, outside interaction with surviving family members. For others, however, their old associations were replaced by new friends with whom it became easier for them to maintain and confirm themselves as now visually impaired. With their new associates they were no longer an old friend proved fallible, no mere 'shadow' of their old selves. Rather, with new associates it became possible for them to build a new shared world within which their visual difficulties were a taken-for-granted part of their personage. Whatever uncertainties the person ever had about giving up the comfort of old friends often gave way to the relative relief of not having to worry any longer about disappoint-

ing them in light of the way things used to be. Goffman notes that
this is common of other stigmatized individuals, observing that
'when the individual acquires a new stigmatized self in life, the
uneasiness he feels about new associates may slowly give way to
uneasiness felt concerning old ones' (1963: 35).

Quite notably, many people who were visually impaired found
themselves developing close relationships with other persons with
visual difficulties. Sometimes this was an unanticipated consequence of the family's urgings for the individual to 'pick up the
pieces' of their life after vision loss. To be accurate, some family
members (especially those of persons for whom the vision loss
occurs while they are still relatively young) eventually begin to
encourage a resumption of life as usual. Not willing to give up
plans for retirement or forgo friendships with other people, several
reported that their spouse encouraged them to resume their active
participation in the world around them after the initial shock over
the loss had passed. Consistent with this goal, they urged visually-
impaired persons to avail themselves of rehabilitation services,
low-vision aids, or any other resources which might assist them in
their struggle to cope with the problems imposed by their vision
loss. One person, for example, insisted that her initial reaction to
stay at home was eventually overcome by her husband's continued
urging that she seek help from various support services. One such
resource was a self-help group for persons with retinitis pigmentosa. The overt purpose of the group was to support one
another through the sharing of common problems, as if to assure
people that they were not alone.

I eventually started going to these retinitis pigmentosa meetings
in [a large city] one winter. Everyone had retinitis pigmentosa
but only in different stages. I was first notified about them by
the Association for the Blind I guess. Well, my husband insisted
that I go. If it had been left to me I'm sure I never would've
gone. I would've stayed at home. But, he insisted that I go. As
it turned out, it was good for me too. We'd shop together and
do different things which made it a fun time. I really think it was
a wonderful thing to go to, because I met the other people and I
figured if they had to cope with it then I certainly could. It gave
me support, you know?

By her own acknowledgement, this individual would not have
made the initial commitment to participate in this group had it not
been for the insistence of her husband. Ironically, however, this
course of action encouraged by her husband (so as to help her re-
embrace her old life and revitalize their mutual friendships) had,

in fact, a somewhat different result. Like so many others who experience new vision loss, while she did eventually become more active in the social arena, her actual network of friends began to change. Increasingly, old sighted friends began to give way to relationships with other couples, one of whose members also shared visual difficulties. This tendency to form new associations with other visually-impaired persons was very common and is deserving of more focused attention.

Interaction with other visually impaired

To a large extent people are able to manage their vision loss by selecting those with whom they interact. As Goffman has observed, often the visually-impaired person is initially put off by other visually impaired in what he calls the 'process of nearing,' i.e. 'the individual's coming close to an undesirable instance of his own kind' (1963: 108). One person, for example, recalled being put off by a 'blind beggar' who used to sit on a corner in the downtown area of his home town. He felt that he demeaned himself by holding out his hat and selling pencils. Another told of what she termed a 'pathetic' blind person who went door to door selling magazine subscriptions and greeting cards. Goffman concludes that this often leaves stigmatized individuals ambivalent about their own circumstance in the light of these other undesirable instances of people sharing their difficulty. Almost every person in this study expressed this sort of initial ambivalence about interacting with other visually-impaired persons. Gradually, however, a large portion of them began to rely upon other visually-impaired persons for the bulk of their intense and emotionally-charged interactions with others. Selecting other visually-impaired persons for this new social network often dramatically alters people's management of their vision loss.

As suggested in the preceding section, often people find themselves associating with other visually-impaired persons as a result of their consumption of available service opportunities – self-help groups, rehabilitation courses, mobility training, etc. In still other instances, there are active local consumer groups which both provide organized leisure opportunities or sometimes provide organized support for issues of particular relevance to visually-impaired persons. The people contacted in this study had such an organization in their midst, though not all were members. In fact, only one-quarter of the people belonged to this group. For them, however, a great deal of their social contacts were enwebbed in the group's activities and friendships growing out of common membership. As it was geared toward both social activities and advocacy for visually-impaired persons, this organization also seemed to fill the social void left by the loss of old friends and family, as well as proved a continuing source of projects which occupied much of their time and planning.

For those who belonged to this local consumer group, fellow members clearly became their 'real group' or the group to which they naturally belong. As Goffman observes, this is again common among persons with some physical disability. He suggests 'the individual's real group, then, is the aggregate of persons who are likely to suffer the same deprivations as he suffers because of having the same stigma' (1963: 113). In Adam Curle's terms, this has significant impact on the person's 'belonging identity,' i.e. their understanding of themselves in terms of 'what they belong to' (1972: 26). One individual succinctly described her natural attraction to her new social network over and against her previous contacts.

> My husband you know works at the plant. Well, they have meetings once a month for supervisors and my husband always goes. Then once a year they have a ladies night. My husband keeps insisting that I will have a good time and he wants me to go. Well, I hesitate to go, you know? Like I tell him, it's different when I'm the only one there that's so inflicted. When I'm with *my* group, you know, there's a lot of others that's in the same boat as I am. So that's different.

The pressure to perform is relieved in a group of people who share a similar loss of vision, know the problems it can create and who take little if any notice when the person falters. As one member of the local consumer group observed,

> I'm comfortable with them. In no time at all I felt close to them. I felt like they were people I could be with and if anything happened it wouldn't bother anyone. You know? They just take everything for granted. I mean you can fall flat on your face and nobody will think 'Oh my!' You know?

Certainly for this reason the organization is very appealing. In addition to this, however, it provides the visually-impaired person with a personal agenda. While Goffman is no doubt correct in observing that such organizations serve to magnify the stigma attached to those persons who belong to the group (1963: 113), it is equally apparent that, for visually-impaired persons themselves, the need to plan for/participate in social activities and various types of advocacy provides them with a new sense of personal direction which supplants the present-oriented approach to life characterizing so many visually-impaired aged individuals. One individual, typical of those belonging to this group, told of how her membership not only provided her with numerous activities but also gave her a sense of belonging and support which made her adaptation to new vision loss much less trying.

I got to the place where I just felt that I had to do something. I just couldn't do it on my own. So I joined the group and I've been with them ever since. I think we're lucky to have this group up here. We're very lucky. It's a nice group of people. Everyone's nice. And you feel like everyone tries to help and that they care, you know, what happens to you. They call up and they say, 'How you doing?' or, 'Is there anything I can do?' They're very considerate. I'm praising them all the time. It's a big help when you get something like this. It's hard to accept it at first, especially when you're alone. I know I couldn't handle it too well. Without the group it would have been harder, I'm sure. I don't think it would have turned out the way it did. They really got me started going out. It really helped a lot. I wouldn't be kind of feeling sorry for myself.

Membership in the group also prompted a number of visually-impaired persons to suggest that it made them feel more influential, people seemed to listen to them more often and their needs were not as likely to be ignored. As one member suggested,

You know politicians, they're always looking for votes. Well if you have an organization it kind of puts pressure on them. And that helps. You know if I go and talk to someone and I just say, 'Hello, I'm Tom Carson,' they'll just think I'm some old guy, you know? But if I say I represent a group of visually impaired persons, you know, they consider you an awful lot more.

In view of their everyday confrontation with powerlessness (their inability to see in the first place, their social dependency upon family and friends, their very inability to fulfill their intentions) it is no wonder that organized visually-impaired persons find this new-found ability to influence the world around them so attractive. It has been suggested by Gaylene Becker (1980) that such consumer-group activities can place the disabled elderly at an advantage over their peers. Many older persons experience late life as a period marked by a decline in personal influence, and the unanticipated power of the group, working for mutually-held interests, can more than offset such losses.

The interaction with other visually-impaired persons in this

78

group context, and indeed even on a more informal basis, also has the effect of helping the person cope with her/his own vision loss cast in relative terms to the losses fellow-members manifest. In Goffman's terms, 'the stigmatized individual exhibits a tendency to stratify his "own" according to the degree to which their stigma is apparent and obtrusive' (1963: 107). Many of the people, both members and non-members of the consumer group alike, often found their own vision loss more digestible in view of the losses of others.

> You know I see other blind people around and that helps. It makes you feel better that you are able to get around a bit better than they can. You almost feel lucky. I know I do. I'm fortunate to see even a little.

Or another:

> I have this blind friend down here and she has a great deal more problems than I have. She has both cataracts and the glaucoma. Then there's another, much younger woman than I am, she has hardening of the arteries, I guess. They don't give her any encouragement. So I've gotten into the habit of counting my blessings against what the rest of them have.

Some members of the local consumer group isolated this reasoning as a moving force behind their enthusiastic embrace of the organization's activities.

> I like to go to all the meetings and to the parties. There are a lot around the holidays. Well you know you meet more friends this way and you see the handicap that someone else has – they're worse off than yourself so you don't feel half so bad that way.

Thus the association with other visually-impaired persons not only creates a social network by which they can maintain their new way of life and provides them, when organized, with a certain sense of power but it also enables them to convince themselves of their relative good fortune in view of the problems other people face. It is seemingly their reverse sense of relative misfortune with their old sighted friends which further pulls them away from the social network which enwebbed them before the onset of their vision loss. Both instances have a marked impact on people's evaluation of their situation which is, of course, important to their very identity in-the-world. As Jervis has noted, the self concept of blind persons depends largely on those they choose for a relative measure (1964: 52).

Coaching

Again, what one comes to know about the world and of experience
is passed on to her/him from others. It is their tried interpretations
of experience by which the world first becomes meaningful.
Information supplied by others is, of course, supplemented by
personal experience with all its trial and error. Yet the world
which is already there and passed on to each social heir remains an
important part of the means by which subjective reality is socially
constructed. One of the most important parts which other visually-
impaired people play in the lives of those experiencing new vision
loss is that of the person who has gone before and who shares her/
his knowledge with those who follow. Any novice relies on the
experience of the expert. Likewise, any candidate for so significant
a physiological change as vision loss finds she/he must rely on the
experience of others who, in turn, stand by quite willingly to
provide the expertise. Anselm Strauss observes,

> Certain aspects of what lies over the horizon are blurred to the
> candidate, no matter how clear his general path. This forces his
> predecessors not only to counsel and guide him, but to prepare
> and coach him beforehand. Coaching is an integral part of
> teaching the inexperienced – of any age. (1969: 110)

Coaching is a critical part of the interrelations between visually-
impaired persons. It is, of course, the guiding principle behind
most of the self-help groups for the visually impaired. Again,
consistent with Strauss' notion of coaching, it would seem that
their efforts revolve largely around attempts 'to move someone
else along a series of steps, when those steps are not entirely
institutionalized and invariant and when the learner is not entirely
clear about their sequences (although the coach is)' (1969: 110).
As one member of a self-help group for persons with retinitis
pigmentosa observed,

> I think it helped me so much to go down to the retinitis
> meetings in Manchester. It was hard for me to go in the first
> place – to admit that I was blind or going to be. Each one down
> there would get up and say different things and tell you what to
> expect. What it would be like. This helped me a great deal.

One aspect of the group's *raison d'être* was to provide a sort of
mapping of what lay ahead and to lend a sort of continuity that
only hindsight could achieve.

The local consumer group also provided a certain amount of
personal coaching. While this was by no means the expressed

purpose of the group, the informal and formal contacts between visually-impaired persons fostered by its organization had this effect. As one member noted,

> I joined the group which really helped me. I could see the others who had lost their sight, you know? How they were handling it and all. They'd talk and I'd listen. I did a lot of listening and I think that really did it for me. That's how I got the upper hand. I'd see somebody else who had the same problem as I did and I could see how they were handling it. They didn't just sit back and feel sorry for themselves. So I thought, 'If they can do it, so can I.'

This informal sharing of experiences was argued to be indispensable by all members of the group. Indeed, several suggested that there was really no substitute for this sharing among people of like circumstance.

> It helps to talk to anybody but I think it's really important to talk with somebody who went through it too. They feel that they are no different. They're on even ground, you know? Yes, I think it's very important that it should be someone that has gone through it. Somebody else might be able to help you but it's not the same.

Most people suggested that while all the coaching in the world could not keep newly visually-impaired persons from going through the various reactions to and frustrations of vision loss, at least this sharing of experiences allowed them to know what to expect and that they were not alone in their experiences.

Those who received this sort of counsel and coaching from their visually-impaired predecessors, seemed to take it upon themselves to pass along their experiences to their successors.

> I've always tried to give a helping hand to people if I could. But today I try even harder – especially with those with poor eyesight. I feel for them a lot, you know, and if there's anything I can do, I go out of my way to do it. I'll call them up on the phone and just talk to them. But you've got to go to them. Not too many will go for help themselves. It takes a little pushing to get them out, you know? By talking through, they're helping themselves.

This person's observations, typical of many members of the consumer group, are distinctively reminiscent of Goffman's remarks regarding the initial support provided by people with other disabilities as well.

> In the case of the individual who has recently become physically
> handicapped, fellow-suffers more advanced than himself in
> dealing with the failing are likely to make him a special series of
> visits to welcome him into the club and to instruct him on how
> to manage himself physically and psychically. (1963: 36)

In a sense, this coaching of others experiencing new vision loss
became a personal mission for several people in this study.
Countless hours were therefore reported spent on the phone
providing guidance and consolation in times of seeming crisis.

Newly visually-impaired persons also receive a certain amount
of indirect coaching from notable role models. These notables may
be universally recognized, such as is the case with Helen Keller.
Susan Dunn (Brooks and Dunn 1974), a 25 year old who became
adventitiously visually impaired, observes that there is a tendency
to look to famous blind persons for a sort of role model.
Accordingly, visually-impaired persons begin to set expectations
and standards for their own adjustment to vision loss. Dunn has
called this the 'Helen Keller syndrome,' and suggests that it
creates a host of additional frustrations when people discover that
they cannot live up to the public image of their disorder. This same
process occurs at the local community level as well, where newly
visually impaired persons often take cues for their own adjustment from the examples set by people in their near environment
whom they deem successful.

> We've got blind people around here – some are teachers,
> lawyers and stuff like that. There's a blind worker with the
> Association for the Blind and she's getting her Master's
> Degree. So you talk to them and you know it can be done.

As 'successful' members of the larger society, quite often then
various professionals who share in vision loss become prototypes
for all those who now find themselves in a similar circumstance.

There are also non-visually-impaired persons who attempt to
coach the person experiencing a new loss of vision. Friends and
family members all have their respective 'Well, if it were me' to
offer. But while the visually-impaired person may listen to their
advice, it is usually discounted as well-intentioned caring of those
who couldn't possibly know what the person is going through.

There is one group of persons that holds a unique place in the
post-visual-loss coaching which most people receive. These are the
people who are in the business of offering the battery of services
which are available to and imposed upon visually-impaired

persons. It would be well beyond the scope of this study to explore the intricacies of the part service providers play in the socialization of the blind. This has been effectively done elsewhere in Scott's *Making of Blind Men* (1969). Several observations are noteworthy, however, in view of their systematic efforts to intervene in people's lives.

While by and large sighted, the people who work with various agencies both specifically and marginally designed to offer services to individuals who are visually impaired are armed with the technological devices, appropriate educational degrees, and organizational structure which makes it possible for them to emerge as *the* experts (see Scott's commentary 1969: 74) in the problems associated with new visual impairment. In the light of their public visibility and often elaborate system of referral programs and community outreach, it is no wonder that most newly visually-impaired persons feel that blindness agencies are the proper agents for their care.

As we observed earlier, all the people in this study had availed themselves of some services from agencies for the blind. This fact automatically excludes those people who have not received such services (most noteworthy perhaps are the hidden or undetected blind) from consideration. For those, however, who seek out agency contacts, the service providers may well signal their first real contact with the world outside their home after their vision loss. For this reason alone, they often play a crucial role in the post-vision-loss adjustment of the aging individual.

Most people indicated that, overall, they felt indebted to and happy with both service providers and the aid they received from them. Indeed, a number credited them with playing a critical role in helping them come to grips with their biological decline. Scott (1969: 74) is no doubt accurate in observing that service providers stress social and psychological rehabilitation rather than medical remedies to vision loss, and many suggested that these same rehabilitative programs prove important as they lure newly visually-impaired persons out of their homes.

I was in sort of a daze for a while after I realized my sight wouldn't get better. It was a shock, you know. Why was this happening? It took me over a year to cope with it. I had to do something with it. Well, the [Blind Service Organization] came up here and offered some classes. I didn't learn anything from the classes but I needed to be there. I needed to do something. So I went and learnt ceramics. I think it was very beneficial to my beginning, to my comeback.

Whether these classes may be judged demeaning or not, it is clear that for the actors themselves they serve as a springboard for getting back to a world of others from the narrow confines of their home. Of course, there is a marked tendency for these new contacts to be with other visually-impaired persons which, in turn, channels activities almost exclusively to those with people who share a similar physiological plight. As has been suggested, this has a profound impact upon the changes which occur within one's social network and correspondingly upon one's very maintenance of subjective identity. Yet the rehabilitation programs of the blindness agencies entice the person out of her/his home and often excite her/his propensity toward resuming interaction with others.

For those persons who have lost many of their friends and family by death, retirement, or institutionalization, the service providers may become the only people they can turn to for support.

It's lucky for me that these people [blindness agency] are up here, 'cause I feel like I can pick up the phone and say I need something. You know, anything. You call up and they're there. It's important to know that somebody's there, somebody that can do something and that cares. You know, you need that reassurance.

For the person left without sight, left without friends and family, 'just knowing someone cares' may provide the minimal reassurance they find so essential for facing day-to-day life.

As Scott suggests, often the initial gratitude gives way to disillusionment and doubt (1969: 75). In part this is due to the fact that they eventually discover that there is actually little that the service providers are prepared to do which will allow them, as older persons, to revive the life they once knew. In part, this is due to the structural limitations imposed by the larger society upon aging persons generally. To a great extent, however, blind services have traditionally made the older visually impaired a relatively low priority. This appears to happen for two reasons:

1　the aged visually-impaired person is seldom totally blind and hence judged not as demanding of attention as are those without any remaining sight; and
2　as Scott has shown, the majority of blind service agencies 'offer a mix of services [which] cater largely to children and non-aged adults who are employable' (1969: 70).

Thus, aged visually-impaired persons discover that they soon exhaust available programs for which they are eligible and become less enthusiastic about those whom they feel have let them down.

Many people reported that they soon became bored with the activities made available to them by the local blindness agency. They were looking for some activities beyond ceramics and basket weaving. One individual likened his treatment by the service providers to that of several bosses he had known while working many years as a city employee.

I've worked for bosses that didn't know what their men could do and all that. You know, if a man is very capable and you give him some little job that's not too interesting, he's going to get bored. You've got to give him something that's challenging. You know, a lot of people will hold you back.

With him, vision loss had resulted in much the same dilemma. There was little training available to him by which he could relearn the skills (both professional and leisure) which had been important to him before the loss of sight. In their stead he found himself working with crafts and feeling that many of those who were supervising his 'rehabilitation' treated him as if he were a 'little child.'

It is in this latter capacity that service providers often contribute to the social dependency discussed earlier in this chapter. Several visually-impaired persons revealed resentment at having so little input into the determination of services made available to them. Correspondingly, they often felt manipulated by service providers. One individual protested, 'I don't have a master's degree but I do have sixty-four years of experience.' Others were outspoken about the very language of dependency which they had grown to resent. Common to many other visually-impaired persons today, they expressed some anxiety over the implicit symbolism conveyed by service providers' use of the term 'client' (a term they found dependency-laden in its symbolic overtones). They expressed preference for the more autonomous term 'consumer.' Consistent with the theoretical premise of this study, this terminological preference demonstrates aged visually-impaired persons' refusal to think of themselves as without input into the very formation and planning of their life course, a task to which they had traditionally been committed.

Social discontinuity and identity

Just as the experience of the body is inseparable from people's ability and indeed their willingness to act out their intentions in the physical world which surrounds them, the experience of and participation in the social world is also an essential part of people's identity-in-the-world. As Berger has suggested, 'self and society are inextricably interwoven entities' (1970: 374–5). People's sense of continuity, situation, and character always takes place within a shared social context. We have, correspondingly, discussed the nature of this shared social world for the aging person experiencing new vision loss.

New vision loss disrupts the person's ability to manipulate the very mechanics of interpersonal communication. Eye contact as a foundational component of successful interaction is, of course, forfeited. So is the ability to digest the series of visual cues which are essential to the give and take of daily conversation. Therefore, the biological decline of the aging eye makes it difficult for individuals to be fully effective in their interaction with others. This, in turn, makes them susceptible to the confirmation of their inadequacy by those around them. This confirmation is often readily forthcoming from even close friends and family members.

There is a marked tendency for those around newly visually-impaired persons to avoid the topic of their vision loss, which quite often gives way to an avoidance of the people themselves. In various interactive settings the person is given a non-person status (to use Goffman's term) and both significant and less significant others will forgo contacts with the visually-impaired person in anticipation of her/his inability to 'hold her/his own' in even the most casual conversation. This anticipation of the person's interactive incompetence is based upon the actual difficulties visually-impaired actors have in managing information in conversational settings (as suggested by the visually-impaired persons themselves) and the virtual social identity which others assign to them (i.e. the imputations of others' sensory problems, etc.).

Family members and friends often provide a sort of protective capsule which insulates the visually-impaired person from many previously-held responsibilities and social involvements. Through their overprotectiveness, significant others generate a feeling of social dependency on the part of the person experiencing new vision loss. As was suggested, this leaves the person feeling powerless to affect the world around her/him. As Scott observes, 'the blind person comes to feel that he is not completely accepted as a mature, responsible person,' and that further, 'as a second class citizen, he must deal with the eroding sense of inadequacy that inevitably accompanies that status' (1969: 37). These feelings of inadequacy have been revealed in this study and have been empirically confirmed elsewhere as well (see Jervis 1964, for example).

Feelings of inadequacy and powerlessness often dissuade visually-impaired persons from seeking out their previous associations with other people. It affects what Argyle (1969) calls the 'motivational' dimension of social competence. It curtails, in other words, people's sheer propensity toward interacting with others. Similarly, as already noted, those people who were once members of a shared social world no longer readily engage the visually-impaired person (note that Scott confirms this observation but discusses its importance in more exchange terms, 1969: 32ff.). Interaction with sighted 'normals' then is often dramatically reduced. Reduced contacts with others flowing from the loss of sight are further exaggerated by shrinkages in the visually-impaired aged person's cohort. These shrinkages are prompted by numerous factors. Friends and family members are placed in nursing facilities, cannot get out because of chronic illness, or may die.

The curtailment of interaction with old friends and family prompted by death, illness, institutionalization, and avoidance often leaves the older visually-impaired person without the very social context within which life used to have meaning. In more traditional sociological language, the older person is often left with a shortage of appropriate reference groups (Rosow 1967; Kuypers and Bengtson 1973). The sensory decline of the body not only makes the navigation of the physical world and the mechanics of social interaction difficult but it also jeopardizes the social relationships of the visually-impaired older person with those by whom she/he mutually maintained and confirmed a shared social world. Again, this erodes a person's 'belonging identity,' i.e. her/his understanding of her/himself in terms of 'what he belongs to.'

Many of the newly visually-impaired actors find themselves increasingly associating with persons who share a similar loss of sight. By availing themselves of services for visually-impaired persons and by joining self-help groups or local consumer groups for people who are blind, they often find their old social network replaced by intense contacts with fellow visually-impaired persons. This contact with others who share their sensory loss helps them forge a new shared social world by providing them with an alternative social environment in which they find themselves, by virtue of their impairment, a natural member. This association with other visually-impaired persons is often quite attractive for several reasons. In the first place, there is a feeling that these people understand the problems they are going through themselves. Secondly, it often provides them with some sense of power which replaces their own powerlessness in interaction with their old sighted world. Perhaps most notably, it provides them with a

sort of apprenticeship to the experience and management of new
vision loss. As Goffman has noted,

> The first set of sympathetic others is, of course, those who share
> his stigma, knowing from their own experience what it is to
> have this particular stigma some of them can provide the
> individual with instruction in the tricks of the trade and with a
> circle of lament to which he can withdraw for moral support and
> for the comfort of feeling at home, at ease, accepted as a person
> who really is like any other normal person. (1963: 20)

Increasingly, then, the newly visually-impaired person comes to
share a world with (also maintained and confirmed by) other
people who have experienced vision loss. The homogeneity of the
visually impaired as a group replaces what was theretofore a number of relatively heterogeneous individuals (Scott 1969: 38).

This process of creating a shared and more homogeneous world
among fellow visually impaired is aided by the intervention of
service providers. As has been noted elsewhere, 'one of the most
important, but least recognized functions performed by organizations of the blindness system is to teach people who have
difficulty seeing how to behave like blind people' (Scott 1969: 71).
Service providers not only bring people of similar sensory losses
together in the first place but they systematically participate in
coaching them. As one of the first major sources of social
involvement outside the home after the onset of vision difficulties,
service providers play a critical role in reshaping people's
experience of the world and themselves. Despite their gratitude to
service providers for supplying them with support at a time when
they often felt abandoned by their old social contacts, many
persons feel that they are manipulated by service professionals and
the latter often contribute to the social dependency that visually-
impaired persons can manifest.

All of the changes which occur in the social life of persons
experiencing new vision loss have a profound impact on their
subjective identity-in-the-world. As Berger suggests, 'to live in the
social world is to live in an ordered and meaningful life' (1967: 21).
This ordering supplies the person with the vocabulary by which
she/he can understand her/his continuity, character, and situation,
her/his identity-in-the-world. To be cut off from one's social world
therefore challenges the in-the-world character of personal identity. Again, Berger asserts

> It is for this reason that radical separation from the social world,
> or anomy, constitutes such a powerful threat to the individual.

It is not only that the individual loses emotionally satisfying ties in such cases. He loses his orientation in experience. In extreme cases he loses his sense of reality and identity. He becomes anomic in the sense of becoming worldless. (1967: 21)

In sacrificing their ties with the world in which they once considered themselves an integral part, people experiencing new vision loss face the threat of becoming worldless. As such their identity-in-the-world is further jeopardized.

Yet people who are visually impaired may begin to 'affiliate' with a new social environment as they simultaneously sacrifice their previous contacts. Matza (1969: 101–2) describes the process of affiliation as 'the adoption or receiving of a son into the family, and by gradual extension, to the uniting or attaching in a close connection those who were previously unattached.' Through affiliation, people learn how to and how not to behave, what is and what is not important. They also learn to accept behavior that would have (prior to affiliation) seemed 'outlandish.' With their sighted social world disrupted, older persons may turn to the host of service providers and the community of fellow visually-impaired others in the hope that these alternative social environments will embrace both them and their loss.

Persons experiencing new vision loss soon discover that their very relationship with both the physical and social world which surround them has been wrenched away. They find that their lives are no longer self evident. On the contrary, their physical and social adventures are now fraught with originary situations each of which demands their assessment, their imagination, and their worry (see Matza's discussion of affiliation as 'conversion' 1969: 104ff.). They are, nevertheless, left with choices; they must select between a variety of possible approaches to their new-found situation and they must choose between a number of anticipated outcomes. Encouraged by a host of service providers, health professionals, and family members, they *may* opt to pursue the enticing shared world with other visually-impaired persons. On the other hand, they *may* decide more or less to withdraw from their previous engagement of the world without replacing it – choosing rather to 'wait out' the remaining years. They *may* even attempt to carry on as if things had not changed. No one of these options necessarily excludes the others and many people will dabble in each. For those who ultimately choose to join the family of visually-impaired persons, to affiliate, there are a number of others (other people who are visually impaired, service providers, etc.) who will help make what at first seems novel become a taken-for-granted part of their sense of themselves. This new life is never unequivocal, however, even for those who begin to reconstruct, maintain, and confirm a new shared world. Rather, they will periodically (some more than others) look back with regret at the life they have forfeited and look forward with doubt at the new world which they have chosen to build (a world they never dreamed they would share).

For most newly visually-impaired people, the changes in their social world which accompany the physical changes in their aging body serve as further reminders that they are now discontinuous from their previously-sighted experience of the world and themselves. It is with this new hold on the world and on their sense of selves that new visually-impaired persons must come to terms. Not only are their senses of ontological security (their sense of themselves as real, alive, and whole) challenged by the physical decline of their biological organisms but they are beleaguered by their acute awareness that their social worlds have been equally altered.

Chapter four
Managing discontinuities of age-related vision loss

Discontinuities of old age

The two preceding chapters have attempted to catalog the impact which new vision loss (accompanying the aging process) has upon people's experience of their bodies and their ability to manipulate the physical and social worlds which surround them and in which they are continually enwebbed. It was suggested at the beginning of Chapter 3 that people's estimations of their situation, continuity, and character are so closely tied to their bodies and the social world that identity is best conceived as identity-in-the-world. Borrowing from Berger and Luckmann (1966: 180), identity can be further argued to be, more specifically, comprised of two ongoing dialectics.

> There is an ongoing dialectic, which comes into being with the very first phases of socialization and continues to unfold throughout the individual's existence in society, between each human animal and its socio-historical situation. Externally it is a dialectic between the individual animal and the social world. Internally, it is a dialectic between the individual's biological substratum and his socially produced identity.

Furthermore, the internal and external dialectics of identity are, in turn, dialectically related to one another. As has been seen, the progressive and often gradual loss of sight disrupts both dialectics; hence it prompts a variety of changes in both the people's relationship to their own bodies and with those significant and less significant others with whom they had shaped an intersubjective world.

Perhaps the central and unifying thread which runs through most of the changes that occur for the person experiencing new vision loss is a theme of loss. Of course the most obvious loss is that of a central sensory skill – the ability to see. Correspondingly, the individual has lost this ability to gather a good deal of the available data about her/his world. The whole of the visual background against which actions in and upon the world are framed is lost. Specific visual cues which are ordinarily taken for granted in communication and which allow the person to navigate through unfamiliar environments become at best suspect. Many objects and others become unknowable to the person who has lost sight.

The loss of sight also prompts the loss of many traditional symbols by which individuals accomplished their very presentation of self. Normal 'hardware,' such as the family automobile, must be sacrificed. The very ability to comport themselves in a manner to which they had become accustomed becomes a daily problematic. Goffman speaks of embarrassing scenes which happen from time to time in everyone's life. As he puts it,

> unmeant gestures, inopportune intrusions and *faux pas* are sources of embarrassment and dissonance which are typically unintended by the person who is responsible for making them and would be avoided were the individual to know in advance the consequences of his activity. (1959: 210)

For newly visually-impaired persons, their very ability to avoid these situations (although they are well aware of their consequences) is lost to them. Rather, unmeant gestures, inopportune intrusions, and *faux pas* become a part of their daily lives.

Many of the activities which were once taken for granted are now unapproachable. One cannot quickly sort through written directions, a book, or a magazine. Leisure activities such as knitting, crocheting, working with wood, or watching television must often be given up. Shopping for daily needs or gifts for others becomes a frustrating affair. Thus, many of the things which comprised a person's daily agenda are seriously disrupted and lost, except when aided by the sighted.

As was indicated in Chapter 3, a person's social network may also be lost. Spouse, friends, and other family members may die. They may be sent to nursing homes. Close friends and family may retire to another area for warmer weather or to be closer to their own family. Severe illness may keep them in their homes. All of these possibilities have the net effect, however, of breaking down the often intense bond between co-participants in a shared social world. These losses beset any older person, but the situation is compounded for the person with new vision loss. Visiting friends who are institutionalized or homebound becomes exceedingly difficult. Often, as has been demonstrated, those friends who remain in the pool of potential contacts avoid visually-impaired persons in anticipation of the awkwardness which might characterize interaction with them.

All of these losses are compounded by the losses which occur because the older person has been removed from various institutional involvements as well. Most have been forced by either their age or their visual difficulty to leave the workplace. Children have long since left home in many instances. They have passed on most of their community activities to succeeding generations. Their institutional context, then, has been curtailed, if not entirely forfeited.

Together these losses form what Shura Saul has called the 'discontinuities' of old age (1983: 44). Saul's choice of wording seems particularly appropriate to describe the losses associated with vision loss, in that these losses raise questions in people's minds as to whether or not they are indeed continuous. Must a person think about her/his relationship to body, things, or others in altogether new terms? It is largely in terms of these losses or discontinuities that a person's sense of situation, character, and continuity is so severely impacted. The individual's continuity is at best equivocal. Her/his situation is indisputably altered. In the face of all that has happened to the physiological and social context, her/his very character is challenged.

It is sometimes difficult for older persons to realize that these losses or discontinuities which do, indeed, impact their sense of situation, continuity, and character are not their 'fault' but that rather they come with the territory of old age. As Rosow has expressed it, 'the losses of old age ultimately overtake everybody, not because they have significantly failed but only because they have survived' (1973: 83). It is not, of course, surprising that people whose lifelong socialization has been steeped in the language of individual responsibility and meritocracy would take such an attitude toward physiological loss as well as career advancement or decline and the like. Regardless of the right- or wrong-headedness of such a cultural tradition, one of the older person's most pressing personal challenges, then, is to make sense of her/his past in the light of her/his present and with a view to the future. The challenge is to discover continuity when often none is readily apparent, to define situation in terms which make it acceptable, and to come to grips with character as at least in some sense still real, alive, and whole. This is the essential problem of age identity-in-the-world.

New vision loss and associated discontinuities beg questions that social scientists have traditionally placed under the heading of 'adaptation,' 'adjustment,' or 'coping.' People who experience the loss of sight in later life certainly find themselves asking 'How do I adapt, adjust, or cope with the challenges posed by vision loss?' They ask themselves 'How will I get along without my old friends?' 'How will I ever manage without my car?' 'How will I shop, cook, and the like?' I am suggesting something different, however, by saying that new vision loss raises the essential problem of age identity-in-the-world. What I mean to suggest here is that people are forced to ask the grander question of 'What does all this mean in terms of my life story, my cumulative sense of who I am?'

New vision loss, in somewhat other words, raises an issue of 'life as narrative' (see, for recent summaries of the approach and its accompanying issues, Bruner 1987; Freeman 1984). People's attempts to answer questions about 'Who am I?' or 'What has become of my life?' find answers through the telling and retelling of their own life stories. Bruner (1987: 11) argues that these stories all people tell about their lives – their 'informal autobiographies' or 'narratives' – must be viewed as evidence of 'world making' as the principal function of mind. Narration is a key part of the interpretive process. Furthermore, the telling of stories has an impact on the way we come to see ourselves and our lives. They are the mechanisms by which people give meaning to sometimes seemingly discrepant life events. Additionally, as Bruner (1987: 15) puts it, 'in the end, we become the autobiographical narratives by which we 'tell about our lives.'

In speaking of 'narrative' or 'life stories' here, I am not speaking of the stories people tell the interviewer. In these instances, the informant reveals glimpses of the life story that becomes part of a personal narrative – a story she/he tells her/himself in an effort to give her/his life meaning. People provide similar glimpses to others around them when they recount key events in their personal development. The stories people tell themselves may be more complex or more detailed than those glimpses they provide to others. Nevertheless, the glimpses can help us understand something of the process by which people deal with age identity-in-the-world. When the person tells her/his story as to why vision loss occurred or why it happened to her/him and not to someone else, we can catalog something of that individual's attempt to give sense to the business of living and to place the loss of the present within the context of past recollections and future anticipations.

The potential outcomes of people's struggle to achieve age identity-in-the-world – that is, the individual's task of making sense of her/his past within the context of the present and keeping the future in mind – has been effectively captured by Erikson's (1980) polar concepts of 'integrity' and 'despair.' Stripped of its psychoanalytic underpinnings, Erikson's conceptual baggage effectively addresses that which becomes so apparent in the experience of people in later life. The outcome of their encounter with the challenges of old age and the narrative patterns they find or fail to find in their lives will take them to either characteristic integrity or despair as they interpret their past, live their present, and anticipate their future. Recalling Erikson's discussion, the person who can be said to have achieved integrity is 'only he who in some way has taken care of things and people and has adapted himself to the triumphs and disappointments of being, by necessity, the originator of others and the generator of things and ideas' (1980: 104). This sense of personal integrity may be counterposed to the sense of despair, or as Erikson puts it 'the feeling that time is too short, too short to attempt to start another life and try out alternative roads to integrity' (1968: 140). Integrity and despair, then, are two alternative outcomes of the older person's efforts to find continuity between her/his recollection of past experience, her/his present, and her/his anticipated future. This effort to find continuity often looks more like a struggle – a struggle to maintain a similar sense of situation and character in the face of an aging body, the inevitable approach toward death, a heavy past, a shortened future, a constricting life/space extensity, and reduced social opportunities. For the person that can face all these things and yet remain 'the generator of things and ideas,' there is characteristic integrity. For the person who finds her/himself unable to apprehend her/his situation, there is the paralysis of despair. Such is the struggle between identity and despair. Let us further explore these two outcomes.

Integrity versus despair in new vision loss

While this struggle between integrity and despair characterizes the lives of all aging persons, it is again brought into relief by the experience of the aging individual experiencing new vision loss. As Rose has observed, 'a change that affects all aging people is the decline in physical powers and the resulting recognition that the incapacities of old age and the nothingness of death are in the inevitable future' (1961: 460). New vision loss makes persons acutely aware of the decline of their physical powers and intimately familiar with the incapacities of old age. The losses and discontinuities so apparent in their lives draw their attention to their physiological decline and their altered relations with physical and social environments. It is no wonder that the struggle between

95

integrity and despair is one with which they are also intimately involved.

For those people who manifested a certain integrity in their lives, the initial shock, anger, and frustrations gave way to a commitment to cope with their difficulties.

Well, like I said, at first I thought I just couldn't get through each day, you know? Do my work or anything. But I found that you've just got to take the bull by the horns and do it. I realized that you couldn't change the situation. You know there are things in this life that you cannot change so you have to learn to live with them. You accept it. That is the hardest thing but if you can accept it you've got it made.

Just as with every other aspect of the experience of new vision loss, people's discovery that they must 'take the bull by the horns' emerges within a social context. Most of those who came to this realization suggested that they did so as much for their family as for themselves. The following example was typical. After months of sitting around her home and having withdrawn from family activities, one person concluded:

It took me a while before I finally decided this isn't doing me or anybody else any good. It wasn't doing me and it wasn't doing my family any good. I'm very close to my family and I didn't want them thinking that it was all over you know? I mean I just decided that I had to shape up. That's all. It was just another problem. Raising my children and my grandchildren there were all kinds of problems and this, I just decided, was just another problem and we'd have to handle it the best we can. That is all you can do about it. Make the most of it, you know? I was glad when that time came. I'll tell you, very glad. I was kind of selfish about my eyes, you know? I thought I was the only one affected. No one else but me. And I thought my family – my husband especially – didn't really care. But then I thought 'Come on now, this is stupid. Wake up! You're putting him through hell too while you're going through it.' I couldn't see keep bringing so much more headache and body ache to my family. It really wasn't fair to them, you know? So I figured it was time for a change.

Her whole system of priorities was impacted by this change from a preoccupation with her own biological decline to a concern with restoring her life in the family. Things would not, of course, be the same as they were before her vision loss but she felt an obligation to reshape her relationship and participation in the family arrangement in ways which would facilitate a normalization of life for everyone concerned.

For those who achieve integrity, there is an often sudden realization that there was really no reason to believe that their lives were any more charmed than others'. Most people suggested that, in their early reaction to vision loss, they could hardly believe that this sensory disruption was actually happening to them. It was one of those things which happen to others but never to oneself. For those who manifested integrity, however, this feeling eventually gave way to a certain acceptance that they were as susceptible to fallibility as anyone else.

You've got to realize that this isn't the end of the line. There are other ways and means of compensating with what you've got. You've got to make an adjustment from one side to another. Sympathy for yourself is one of the worst things in the world for you. I mean I think this is what we all do – you feel sorry for yourself. You say, 'Why me?' Well, why not you? You know? That's what it comes down to.

Increasingly, persons who arrive at integrity begin to 'count their blessings.' As Butler observes, 'reviewing one's life . . . may be a general response to crises of various types' (1968: 488) and the confrontation with new vision loss seems to be consistent with his claim. Yet people can choose to look back on their pasts with regret or with a certain sense of fulfillment. Clearly, no person ever feels that she/he has achieved everything she/he set out to do. For most, Yeats' suggestion that 'life is a long preparation for something that never happens' (quoted in de Beauvoir 1972: 491) seems to ring with a certain truth. For those who have adapted themselves to life's triumphs and disappointments, however, their life review places their vision loss within the context of their life's whole.

I had a happy childhood. I had good parents and a good family life. And after I was married, I was lucky. I had a good husband. And like I tell my sons 'I don't want to go blind but I've had a good life. I've had a good marriage. I've good boys and I've got grandchildren' and I says 'I've got good memories so I don't have any kick coming.'

As another person recommended 'you've got to look on the bright side of things.'

Well, I always did say that if you could laugh or make light of some things I think it's a lot better than looking down on everything. Look at the good side of it, you know? I feel as though I've had a very fortunate life. I mean, I've had ups and downs like everyone else. Maybe a few more than some and maybe a few less than some. But I've had a very lucky life. I think I've been very fortunate, you know? Healthwise and everything else. So why complain?

This, coming from a woman who at 57 years of age can no longer identify colors, read, or recognize the features of family members' faces and who had lost one leg in an amputation prompted by the same diabetes which had taken her sight, signals the integrity of a person who has come to terms with her own biography. She, like others, embodies the meaning of integrity in the face of the aging process.

Those persons who have achieved integrity typically treat their organismic decline as something which comes with the territory of aging. Again, they do not see themselves set out as the target of some unexplainable punishment but rather see themselves as experiencing the trappings of old age.

It's my age, you know? You don't gain too much sight with age, anyway. I don't know if glaucoma is a disease or what. It's something that happens to your body. It's not a germ or anything like that. It's a malfunction. But with age you accumulate these things. I know that.

Some insist that it is this realization which makes the loss of sight so much easier to accept.

I think in a much younger person – I think it means so much more. And well I guess in the older person it does but it doesn't. I mean, we may wonder what we're going to do, who's going to see to us and all that but at the same time, I would say that an older person has the will to accept things more. I think about the only way to tell you is that you've got to learn to accept it. If it is to be it will be. You can't worry because that's the way it is with everything near the end.

For the person who has attained integrity, then, organismic decline is recognized as the price of survival. There is no need to sort through one's past in search of a reason for vision loss. It is one disruption among others which can beset the aged cohort.

For some older persons, aging clearly has remained a daily problematic with which they have been unable to come to terms. Those persons tend to feel as though they have been singled out for their personal trial. Their difficulty is not simply one amongst the others which beset persons who share in their old age. They continue to ask the question 'Why me?' In Erikson's terms, they are prone to despair. As he further suggests, such persons often hide their despair behind 'a show of disgust, a misanthropy, or a chronic contemptuous displeasure with particular institutions and particular people' (1980: 105).

In sharp contrast with the resolve manifested by the diabetic individual who had lost both her sight and her leg, another visually-impaired person with diabetes offered the following assessment of her circumstance:

> I sure see a lot of people on the street that I would like to change places with. Oh yes, they seem to be able to do everything. I mean I'm not that old that I should be tied down with a lot of things, you know? But that's what I get for cheating. I gotta awful sweet tooth. I guess all diabetics do. They crave something sweet.

This search of the past for some personal failing (to explain the loss of vision) seems characteristic of those persons who despair. Rather than seeing their problem as characteristic of their age cohort, they look for some precaution they failed to take or some abuse they were unable to avoid. Their search often leaves them bewildered and confused. This bewilderment is further compounded by their observation of 'less deserving' persons who have managed to avoid the calamities of old age. As one person bitterly complained,

> I keep asking myself why would it happen to me when I have always taken care of myself and I enjoy everything, doing everything? Then I think of all the people around the world that oh, I see some downtown, you might call them bums – who seem to have perfect eyesight. So why did it happen to me?

Rather than 'taking the bull by the horns' or 'looking on the bright side' or 'making the best of things', the person who experiences despair sees few ways to bring their life back into the unproblematic. Rather than seeking to restore some order to their lives, they either resolutely 'wait for their call' (as one individual put it) or they almost seem to want to hurry the end along.

> My greatest hope is to drop dead. Would you believe that? There is nothing I would like better than to drop dead. I don't want to be a demand on anybody. That's why I'd like to drop dead. I haven't got a hell of a lot of money but I'd give it all if I knew I was going to drop dead. What the hell is the use of

living? Tell me. What have I got to look forward to? You can't answer that, can you? No, you can't. Just another day. That's all.

As Butler and Lewis observe, 'reactions to death are closely related to a resolution of life's experiences and problems as well as a sense of one's contribution to others' (1977: 40). They have noted, therefore, that it is common for terminally-ill patients to 'welcome' death as they begin to experience more pain and feel less and less a part of their family's life. In a similar sense, some of those persons with new vision loss began to view death as much less threatening in the light of the problems their vision loss caused them, their relative incapacity, and the collapse of their social network. These people fully understood the meaning of Erikson's concept of despair. Indeed, they knew full well that it was too late for them to seek out 'alternative routes to integrity.'

Very few people manifested a constant state of despair. Rather, it was common that they would vacillate between integrity and despair throughout their day-to-day experience and within the interview situation itself. As one 77 year old reported,

There are so many things you can't see. In a way I should be really depressed. You know what I mean? I try to build myself up and then all of a sudden I'll start to cry, you know, and I say 'You can't do that.' 'I better stop.' 'I'm not going to pity myself.' 'I'm not going to baby myself.' 'I'm going to be a strong person.' 'I'm going to bear it.' But then again, in two hours or so, it gets to me again.

Even those people who are busily attempting to come to terms with the world around them find themselves vacillating between integrity and despair in those moments when they sit back and reflect on their circumstances.

It's not good to just sit there and think of it and worry about it. It won't make it any better. Of course, I'm not that brave. I can't say that some nights I don't think about it. I worry and get kinda scared. You know? But I get over it and say 'Well, tomorrow's another day' and I do the best I can. It's only when I'm not too busy. If I have things to do and I am kept busy, I won't think about it. It is only when I have time on my hands. Like at night, I won't be going out and I'm just sitting there and I start thinking about it. I say 'My gosh, is this really happening?' You know?

Many people suggested that they had a lot of 'time on their hands'

– moments when they find themselves unoccupied and thinking about their vision loss and how things used to be confront them all too frequently. In those moments, even those who have more or less come to terms with life's triumphs and disappointments will acknowledge feelings (however fleeting they might be) of self-doubt and worry at what additional problems the future holds.

For those older persons who have achieved integrity, these feelings seldom occur in relation to their overall embrace of life, past, present, and future. For those persons more closely approaching despair than integrity, these feelings pervade a much larger part of their lives. For the latter, their problems often become the paramount concern of their daily agenda. They dwell upon the failing of their body, the loss of their friends and family, and thus convey a sense of having been betrayed in both their physical and social experience.

Roads to integrity

Now that some of the characteristic self-appraisals of those who achieve integrity or dwell in despair have been outlined, the question arises: How is it that some people achieve integrity and still others are left preoccupied with their own despair? Many of those who seemingly had come to terms with their new visually-impaired way of life offered the explanation 'time heals everything.' Indeed, time did play a major role in distancing people from the initial shock and disbelief of their new vision loss. Time seemed a necessary part of achieving integrity, but it certainly was not (in and of itself) a sufficient explanation. There were those who had achieved integrity within one year of the onset of their visual difficulties and those who ten years later were still steeped in personal despair. What, then, combined with the passage of time to facilitate the integration of their present crisis with their past accomplishments and disappointments and their admittedly uncertain future?

As alluded to earlier, those people who were able to achieve integrity seemed to demonstrate a unique capacity to retain continuity with their recollected past and anticipated future. This is not to say that they felt the same toward their body or toward their social world. Not one of the people that I interviewed would have made this claim. Their lives were a latticework of discontinuities and losses, as discussed earlier. Continuity rested, however, in their ability to treat their vision loss as one more of life's personal events. As such, new vision loss required the same attitudinal mechanisms which allowed them to survive previous life crises and which they felt confident would allow them to deal with any other problems in the future.

In spite of the apparent discontinuities in their lives (organismic and social), those persons who discovered integrity found that certain attitudes sedimented in their past experiences allowed them to confront aging and vision loss as well. One individual, for example, likened his personal resiliency in coping with new vision loss to his adaptability in past work experiences.

> I worked for a boss one time, he didn't last long, only ten months. Boy, I never despised a man that much before. At the time I was working in the shop – taking care of gasoline and oil in the cars, greasing and the tires, everything. Tire changing for the snow and all that. Well, every morning when he'd come in the first thing of all he'd drive up to the pump for some gas and he'd say 'Wipe my car.' He'd make me wipe that damn car every day. Every day it had to be wiped and cleaned up. And that's a job I hated to do. And it was the way he'd ask – he'd tell me to do it. But I'd do it. I'm not hard to adjust. I can adapt myself to almost anything.

It is, in part, this attitudinal continuity with past experiences that allows individuals to cope with the experience of biological and social fallibility. They discover some sense of sameness in the face of the multiplicity of discontinuities their vision loss otherwise imposes upon them.

Buoyed by the successful outcomes of past experiences, persons who achieved integrity viewed their vision loss (and even aging itself) as a sort of challenge akin to those already handled so well.

> I don't give up, you know? This is the way I've always done things. I'm not one to sit down and just wait for things to happen or have somebody else do things for me. I've just gotta do things. Once I set my mind on something it's, well, it's kind of hard to change. I had smoked for years and tried to stop many times. But I knew that I had to decide when I'd stop smoking. Well, one day I got up and I said 'That's it. I'm not smoking anymore.' And I never did. If I set my mind to something, that's it.

This person, like others, had 'set her mind' to adjusting to vision loss as well. The result was that she made a concerted effort to overcome the frustrations it imposed and sought out new acquaintances who would supplant the ones she had lost. She believed that her determination had enabled her to stop smoking, and she further believed that it would similarly carry her through the difficulties imposed by the loss of sight.

A certain continuity with the past is also gleaned from the knowledge that others had made it through similar vision loss before. There is a sort of continuity with one's predecessors in vision loss.

> Why feel depressed about it or feel sorry for yourself? There is nothing to be done. And I say to myself 'I'm not the first person who's been blind and I'm not going to be the last person who will be blind.' So I don't like it but I'm going to accept it. If they could do it, I can, that's what I believe. If the next person can – I can try.

People's own success in coping with various life crises are, then, supplemented by the experiences of their predecessors. Both fortify their commitment to adapt to the problems of vision loss. As the discontinuities of bodily experience and changing social network become ever increasingly apparent, people who achieve integrity put emphasis on their attitudinal continuity in the face of adversity and the ancestral continuity they share with other visually-impaired persons gone before.

For the person who faces old age and new vision loss with integrity, this search for both personal and shared continuity not only reaches back to the past but extends toward the anticipation of the future as well. Indeed, it is the fear of the future – more specifically, the fear of the additional losses which the future will bring – that often plunges the person toward despair. The following response typifies the more intense despair this fear of the future can evoke.

> You know now I've got a little bit of sight on the sides. If I look sideways I can still see a little of what I'm doing. Which is a hell of a lot, I'm telling you. Jesus, if I had to go – I'd hate to go – I'd want to die before I'd go blind. It must be terrible. I've suffered like hell already but I wouldn't have the guts for that.

It is the anticipation of a future life of total blindness and the inability to cope with even the thought of that eventuality which often leads visually-impaired persons to despair about their present. Even those who have found some sense of attitudinal continuity, linking their past crises with the vision loss of their present, begin to despair when they look toward the future and the anticipation of total blindness. These people hold the belief that the sedimentation of their past experiences would be grossly insufficient to deal with that development. One person, for example, reported that she had found that her life had prepared her 'to handle almost anything that comes up.' Yet when she contemplated the future she began to slip toward despair.

If I only could be certain that my sight had reached a point where that's it, you know? I wouldn't lose anymore. But you just lose a little bit more of your sight as you go along and you keep wondering how bad it's going to get. I'll think about that. I'll wake up during the night and think about it. It still happens all the time. You say 'How bad will it get?' Then you start worrying about how bad it can get. You start thinking panicky. You think about going completely blind. That's the thing. If it was a sure thing that you would keep some of your eyesight then you wouldn't worry about it too much.

While most people were advised by various medical professionals that they would never go completely blind, those who slipped toward despair found such counsel of little comfort. They feared rather the final discontinuity which total blindness threatened, the discontinuity represented by their anticipated inability to come to terms with the complete loss of sight.

Those persons who seemingly achieved the greatest sense of personal integrity in the face of aging and vision loss projected an approach to life which allowed them to integrate past with present difficulties on to the future as well. They were confident that they would be able to adjust to life's challenges in the past and they anticipated this same outcome in the face of future losses. In a sense, they were able to get beyond the early preoccupation with the vivid present. As one person noted (when asked about her anticipation of additional loss of sight),

I will just accept it. If it is to be it will be and there's nothing I can do about it so I will accept it and make the best of it. I can't cry.

Another individual, contemplating future losses, insisted,

If I can't see as good I will just have to learn something else. I can't sit here and do nothing. If I become blind I know I won't be able to do what I've been doing. You know? I will just have to put everything aside and learn something else. I will be frustrated for a while but I will work it out of my system. What God hands out I will have to take.

The road to integrity, then, is marked by the person's ability to take new vision loss as one more of life's challenges. This challenge is linked to the past by the recollection of effective resolutions to crises gone by and to the future by belief that 'I can do it again,' no matter what the future brings.

Furthermore, persons who exhibited integrity in their handling of aging and new vision loss were characteristically able to place their own losses in relation to those of others. (As suggested earlier, this ability to contextualize their losses is an earmark of integrity.) The 'time that heals' is often spent contextualizing one's losses within the pool of potential losses experienced by others in the aged cohort. Such contextualization requires not only the time since onset but the years preceding it which were spent in watching others face life's adversities.

> You more or less learn to live with what you have, I think, over the years. Or else you're unhappy if you don't. I never could see this nagging or complaining because there is nothing you can do about it. Why not accept it and say 'Well, God was good to me after all'? I'm able to do a lot more than these people you see in wheel chairs and things like that. It's better to go with a cane than a wheel chair. If you want to look around you see so many others so much worse off than you are. If you don't believe me, you go up to the nursing home up here. When you come back you'll be so thankful you're able to do all the things you do do. No, I won't complain. Regardless of what happens.

Or as another suggested,

> By thinking of others, that helps you. You look around you and you say 'Well, look at the problems they have' you know? Or you say 'Well, I'm lucky I don't have that problem.'
> Everybody's got their share and their load to carry and all that. If it's not one thing then it's another. So me, I don't consider myself unfortunate.

Interestingly enough, a number of people who were able to so locate themselves within the misfortunes of their fellows in aging exhibited a certain impatience with those who chose to despair.

> You got to live with things no matter what it is. Whether it's a heart ailment or anything else. Why if you have an impairment, you have to live with it. Some people worry themselves to death over some things, you know? Don't worry me so much though. I get irritated seeing people all the time who say 'Oh, I'm in terrible pain' and they're actually the picture of health, you know? They got a rheumatic twinge or something like that and that's all. But they're always talking about it. Me, I'm a fellow that takes things as they come.

In integrity, then, persons accept their own difficulties as the 'load' they were destined to carry, over and against the loads carried by others. It is, as Erikson observes, 'the acceptance of one's one and only life cycle . . . as something that had to be and that, by necessity, permitted no substitutions' (1968: 139). The load is easier to carry, however, in the realization that 'it could have been worse.' Fortunately, it is always possible to construct, if only in hypothetical terms, a worse situation than the one in which a given person finds her/himself. Thus, the road to integrity can be traversed by persons with a wide range of personal difficulties and is restricted only by the limitations of an individual's ability to contextualize her/his circumstance.

Berger has argued that one of the most effective means for coming to terms with 'marginal situations' (i.e. 'situations in which he [the individual] is driven close to or beyond the boundaries of the order that determines his routine, everyday existence,' Berger 1967: 23) is the application of 'theodicies.' Theodicies are explanations or justifications, in religious terms, for human suffering (Berger 1967: 53). They take on varying degrees of sophistication. Those of concern at present are utilized by the actors themselves in their effort to make sense of their own personal suffering and misfortunes. A number of people that I spoke with attempted to make sense of their misfortune, their suffering, through religious expressions which allowed them to place their vision loss within the context of an overarching sacred canopy. People would use such phrases as 'You must count your blessings,' 'We all have our cross to bear,' or 'Whatever is God's will will be.' These commonsensical (that is, without pronounced theological sophistication) theodicies seemed to enable persons not only to contextualize their losses with those of others but also enabled them to intertwine their own problems within a sacred frame of reference. Geertz notes that the religious problem of,

> suffering is, paradoxically, not how to avoid suffering but how to suffer, how to make physical pain, personal loss, worldly defect or the helpless contemplation of others' agony something bearable, supportable – something, as we say, sufferable. (1973: 104)

Those persons who achieved integrity in the face of their worldly defect of new vision loss often turned toward such commonsense theodicies to help make their new life sufferable.

Perhaps the most striking feature of those people who seem to have achieved integrity in their aging and vision loss is the sustained commitment they demonstrate to living in the world.

This is to say that they continue, despite their biologically- and socially-imposed limitations, to engage the world around them. The world to which they find themselves committed is, of course, changed in many ways. It is a world absent of much of the normal hardware they once knew and it is filled with deviant hardware which plays an increasingly important part in their daily lives. It is a world in which activities once taken for granted have become exceedingly difficult to accomplish. It is a world of reduced sensory information. It is a world in which old significant others and the chorus of casual contacts may play less important parts. In spite of these changes, persons who have achieved integrity find ways to sustain their commitment to others and to action in and upon the world (no matter how drastically changed that world may be).

Having contextualized their losses and come to terms with life's triumphs and disappointments, persons who achieve integrity begin to re-carve a personal agenda, reform social ties, and revitalize their dedication to mastering the challenges each day presents. As one person advised those facing vision loss,

It is there. You can't run away from it. So the best thing to do is to face it. It's hard – I'm not saying it's easy – it's very hard. It takes different lengths of time for different people. But you can't just sit. You've got to accept it and after that's done, then you've got to get on your way and do things. Do things you like, not force yourself to do things you don't care for. If you are interested, you'll like it. Yes. Do it.

The earlier-cited diabetic 57-year-old woman who showed her integrity in the face of severe visual loss and the amputation of her leg clearly demonstrated this commitment to remain engaged with the world. Her resolve was borne out not only in her handling of her vision loss but also in the management of her artificial limb. As she reported,

They [her family] don't believe that I will be able to put up with all this. I know I can. I had my leg amputated and the worst part was when I got my new leg. I told them it was a fat leg and didn't look like mine at all. I didn't like it so I threw it in the car. My boys came over and they said 'Ma, this isn't like you.' Well, when I was alone with nobody around I would go to my room and put it on and hobble around. The first thing I knew, I kept it on all day. I gotta keep pushing.

Her desire to 'keep pushing,' like so many others who achieve integrity, helped her maintain her involvement in her family's affairs, to forge new friendships, and ultimately to grapple with the severe disruptions to her bodily experience.

The desire to remain committed to the world and to others seems to flow, at least in part, from a desire to retain a certain sense of personal autonomy; to be, in Erikson's words, the originator of things and ideas. Persons who achieve integrity find a balance between their necessary dependence upon the cooperation of others and their struggle to remain an independent originator of the world around them.

> Some people sit in their chairs all day and feel sorry for themselves all the time. Self pity, you know? They want everybody to do something for them. I don't. I can't accept that. I don't want nobody to baby me. When I need help, I holler.

The world in which they are the originator may be very different in some ways from the world they once knew and in which they participated. They may not be able to do all the things they once did and the people with whom they reaffirm their mutual sense of situation may be different, but nevertheless they remain actors in the full sense of the word. They are not the passive recipients of a world, but rather act upon it to give it meaning.

To achieve integrity, then, people may re-define their sense of physical and social life space (Clark and Anderson 1967: 398ff.). They may alter their perception (as a realistic response to their circumstance) of space and time. They may experience changes in the people who maintain and confirm their sense of self. In the end, however, they manage to interpret their present in view of their past and future, and they remain embedded in a social network which gives their life a shared quality. They realize, in de Beauvoir's terms, that

> There is only one solution if old age is not to become an absurd parody of our former life, and that is to go on pursuing ends that give our existence a meaning – devotion to individuals, to causes, social, political, intellectual or creative work.
> (1972: 540)

Integrity – the transcending of individuality

In sum, the capacity to achieve integrity in the face of new vision loss and other discontinuities of the aging process seems to rest in the person's ordering of experience which transcends her/his own unique problems and circumstance. People, in other words, transcend their individuality. Each of the various roads to integrity discussed above represents a particular strategy by which this transcending of one's own problems, one's own pain, one's own fear of the uncertain future ahead can be achieved.

The capacity to transcend one's own triumphs and disappointments is facilitated by the various experiential strategies outlined above. By turning to religious theodicies, for example, the person is able to place her/his own experience within a sacred frame of reference. It comprehends people and all their experiences, including those of their visual difficulties, the disruption of their social world, the challenges to their sense of space and time, and even the impact of these changes on their sense of situation, continuity, and character. In other words 'these events are now given a "place" in the scheme of things which constantly is protected from the threat of chaotic disintegration that is always implicit in such events' (Berger 1967: 59).

Yet this same transcendence can be facilitated by other experiential strategies which do not rely on sacred validation. People can transcend the problems of the present by searching for a continuity with their recollected past and their anticipated future. While new vision loss seems to lead people to focus inordinately on their present, people effectively transcend this fixation on their present by seeking an overview of their experiential whole. They transcend their present, in other words, by finding a certain attitudinal continuity that links their present visual difficulties with their past triumphs and disappointments and the anticipation of future challenges and resolutions. Vision loss and the additional discontinuities it carries with it become part of the ongoing flow of personal events that together constitute a person's biographical experience. In achieving such an experiential overview, people transcend or come to view their lives as wholes (a totality) rather than focusing on any of life's disparate biographical events (including, and most notably, their present visual difficulties).

Similarly, persons with new vision loss transcend their own problems of the present by coming to view their difficulties as shared with others of like circumstance (predecessors, contemporaries, and heirs). To recall the remarks of one person cited earlier in this chapter, 'I'm not the first person who's been blind and I'm not going to be the last.' People can transcend their often profound sense of personal difficulty by viewing themselves as part of a greater social whole – a whole whose parameters are defined by the visual declines in which they share. This realization that they are part of many like-affected persons may, of course, take organizational form in visually-impaired persons' participation in consumer groups, self-help groups, and other social arrangements which systematically confirm for them that they are not alone.

Finally, visually-impaired persons can transcend their present-oriented focus on their problems by restoring a commitment to the world. This commitment may often be temporarily misplaced by new vision loss and its interrelated physical and social discontinuities. If it is restored, if persons rekindle their hold on experience as a physiological, social, and psychological whole, then it is quite possible that they can loosen the hold of despair and turn toward the task of remaining, by necessity, the originator and generator of things and ideas.

In essence, then, transcending individuality is accomplished by restoring or maintaining the full dialectical interplay of what is identity-in-the world. This unity of individual, biological organism and shared social world must be successfully maintained if one is both to transcend her/his individuality and, hence, to achieve integrity in the face of the discontinuities of the aging process. Only those people who come to terms with the intentional unity of their lives, their projects, their relevances in relation to their changing bodily experiences and shifting social environments will be able to view their own suffering and misfortune as encompassed by some greater whole (the whole of their life course, the whole of fellow blind, the whole of some cosmic agenda) and thereby traverse the road to integrity.

To recall the remarks of Berger *et al.* (1973: 63), 'to be human . . . is to live in a reality that is ordered and gives sense to the business of living.' New vision loss, as one of many discontinuities which accompany old age, challenges the meaningful ordering of reality in ways that have been outlined in great detail. It may push the people toward the boundaries of order which make their everyday existence meaningful. As such, it is clearly one of many marginal situations which confront older persons. For the individual to come to terms with this indisputably personal event, it is necessary for her/him to somehow surrender her/himself to some greater interpretive scheme which subsumes her/his own individual experience. By doing so, 'his birth, the various stages of his biography and finally his future death may now be interpreted by him in a manner that transcends the unique place of these phenomena in his experience' (Berger 1967: 54). In this way people can achieve integrity.

The social context of integrity

As one reflects on the stories of those people who confront vision loss, there is a tendency to conclude that the struggle between integrity and despair is a matter of one individual's personal courage, inner strength, or resolve compared to the relative lack of these characteristics in another. To be sure, people displayed courage, strength, and resolve, but these traits can be found in both those who achieve integrity as well as those who are left with despair. It would also be a mistake to 'blame the victim', if you will, for failing to achieve integrity – for failing to make sense of her/his life in terms of some greater whole. The characteristically human enterprise of sense-making is not something that is undertaken individually. It is a fundamentally collective or social process. As such, we must remind ourselves that the roads to integrity always cross a social landscape, not solely a psychological one.

Each of the strategies that people use to place vision loss within some larger context emerge in and out of shared interaction with others. Again, it is clear that people can effectively place their losses within a sacred frame of reference by utilizing theodicies. Yet the use of commonsense theodicies is suggestive of something more than personal spirituality. In large part, theodicies are a matter of legitimation. As Berger defines it, legitimation means '*socially objectivated* "knowledge" that serves to explain and justify the world order' (1967: 29, italics added). Legitimations of any sort, in other words, are not of any one individual's making: rather, they are part of the cultural baggage that is made available to people by virtue of their membership in a society. They are part of the language system that people inherit socially. By saying that legitimation is 'objectivated,' Berger is correctly asserting that people are aided by socially-supplied explanations in their quest to supply some meaning to the existing world order, whether that world order refers to the unequal distribution of wealth or disabilities. This socially-objectivated knowledge can take place at a variety of levels – religious justifications, or theodicies, being one. At another level is the use of proverbs, moral maxims, and the like. This form of legitimation is also apparent among those experiencing vision loss. Expressions such as 'you have to look on the bright side,' 'count your blessings,' or 'make the best of things' all guide people in their attempts to make sense of their situation. More to the point here, however, is the fact that such expressions are passed on to the individual by others. The road to integrity is not only suggestive of the basic human insistence on finding order in life; it is also suggestive of the fact that our sense-making capacity and our personal narratives – the very ways in which we tell and order our life stories to and for ourselves (as well as others) – are socially derived.

This same point can be made with regard to people's attempts to place their own loss of eyesight within the context of all those other people who have experienced vision loss. For those people who find themselves members of a new 'real group' – a group of like-situated persons experiencing vision loss – the social nature of realizing that 'I am not alone in my loss' is quite apparent. Through formal programs and informal counseling among members, those who join consumer groups find comfort in belonging, a language for telling their story, and assurance that vision loss did not befall them alone. Furthermore, there is a sort of social vindication that seems to accompany group membership. If similar losses can befall fellow members – who they come to know as equally undeserving of their 'lot' – then the need to search the past for some personal failing becomes less urgent. This same social vindication can be found outside the consumer group as well. As pointed out earlier, some people are able to locate their vision loss within the greater pool of all potential losses that come with old age. They can compare (often favorably) their loss of sight with stroke victims, people who have lost hearing, etc. People find comfort and indeed personal vindication in learning that 'bad things' or even 'worse things' happen to those they judge to be 'good people.'

People's decision to re-commit themselves to an involvement in the world also occurs within a social context. For those people who experience a sort of 'protective encapsulation' by members of their families, a sustained commitment to the world in which they had been involved in the past becomes more difficult. To commit oneself to the world requires a view of one's own reality that allows a place for such commitment. 'It "really" is possible for me to pursue my goals and projects.' Such views of reality require the support of others if they are to be successfully maintained or even imagined.

> Worlds are socially constructed and socially maintained. Their continuing reality, both objective (as common, taken-for-granted facticity) and subjective (as facticity imposing itself on individual consciousness), depends upon specific social processes, namely those processes that ongoingly reconstruct and maintain the particular worlds in question. Conversely, the interruption of these social processes threatens the (objective and subjective) reality of the worlds in question. Thus each world requires a social 'base' for its continuing existence as a world that is real to actual human beings. This 'base' may be called its plausibility structure. (Berger 1967: 45)

If a person is separated from the 'social base' (her/his institutional involvements, associations with others, etc.) upon which she/he built a sense of reality, then the world as she/he knows it becomes less plausible and it becomes more difficult to maintain her/his place in it. The parameters of the world the person considers to be her/his own, plans, and even self-estimations become problematic when the 'plausibility structure' is lost or changed significantly. Protective encapsulation can certainly diminish a person's plausibility structure to this end. Alternatively, strategies that maximize a person's commitment to a firm social base, a plausibility structure, may similarly encourage a continued commitment to the world. As Berger has also pointed out, this issue of plausibility structure is related to the issue of legitimation that was raised above. 'The firmer the plausibility structure is, the firmer will be the world that is "based" upon it.' Conversely, 'the less firm the plausibility structure becomes, the more acute will be the need for world-maintaining legitimations' (Berger 1967: 45).

While emphasizing the social context of the roads to integrity, it is important that one refrain from assuming any unidirectional causality. Throughout our lives we are constrained by the relationships that we have with other people. In this sense, we can speak of the 'determination' of our lives. All people experience social 'boundedness' by virtue of the social control that significant others as well as institutions exert upon them. Yet people cannot be understood as mere receptors of social determination. As actors, they have a capacity to act back.

> Unlike all other beings in the empirical world . . . human beings are capable of doing and thinking genuinely new things. This capacity is necessarily linked to the capacity of saying no – be it to supernatural forces, to the forces of nature, to one's own body, and of course to all aspects of society. Man can only be free by saying no, by negating, the various systems of determination within which he finds himself or (using the language of existentialism) into which he has been thrown. Man's freedom only makes sense if it implies this transcendence of causalities. (Berger and Kellner 1981: 96)

Berger correctly reminds us that to recognize simultaneously that people are 'free' (in the sense he describes) and yet live within systems of determination is not contradictory. Both 'perceptions' are 'applicable to the same phenomena.' Stuart Charme (1984) suggests that Jean-Paul Sartre equates human 'consciousness' with 'choice' for much the same reason.

> Sartre equates 'consciousness' with 'choice' to distinguish it from genuine deterministic processes that operate in the physical world. Consciousness is discontinuous with deterministic mechanisms because they fail to account for the power of consciousness to transcend the conditioning factors of any situation. (Charme 1984: 25)

The point here is that the social contexts within which the struggle between integrity and despair take place cannot be used to predict unfailingly how one person versus another will make sense of vision loss. The fact that theodicies are made socially available to people does not mean that all people will find them useful or will activate their legitimating power. The self-help ideology of consumer groups will not automatically enable a person to recommit her/himself to the various life projects that she/he pursued before vision loss, nor necessarily provide her/him with a new agenda. The protective encapsulation of the family does not inevitably leave a person without a 'social base' for maintaining a sense of reality. One can say 'no' to theodicies and other forms of legitimation, one can say 'no' to the ideology of the consumer group, one can say 'no' to the protectiveness of the family. By the same token, these various 'systems of determination' cannot be ignored. They cannot be wished away. They define the options that are readily available, they make one choice easier than another and they provide a language that may or may not be conducive to understanding the whole of one's life story. But then this is the necessary ambiguity that results from the dialectical nature of human identity (as outlined at the beginning of this chapter) and this is precisely why the social environments within which self-understanding, human actions, and choices occur are best thought of as contexts and not causes.

Chapter five

Maintaining self and reality in late life

The moment has arrived to take stock of the discussion over the preceding chapters. A good deal of theoretical and empirical landscape has been traversed and as such the task of this last chapter lies primarily in providing an integrative overview which will, hopefully, punctuate the central thesis of the study. Beyond this, however, the lessons provided by age-related vision loss regarding aging and the even broader issue of human experience must be considered. There are a number of questions that can guide our discussion here. To begin, we must ask: What do the narrative stories that have been reviewed here tell us about how we should theoretically understand and articulate vision loss, aging, and identity? Likewise we must ask: What does aging and new vision loss tell us about the experience of other physical and social changes associated with later life? Finally, we must consider: What does it tell us about human experience more generally?

Aging and new vision loss: an overview

As characterized in the preface, the study can be best understood as an inquiry into people's experience of themselves as they confront striking reminders of their changing bodies, changing social relationships, and even the finite nature of their existence in the world. While it specifically investigates the loss of sight in later life, it is, more broadly understood, an attempt to develop the interrelationships between subjective identity and the aging process.

Vision loss 'explodes' the taken-for-granted nature of people's relationship to and understanding of both their bodies and their ties to other people. As such it also challenges people's sense of themselves as 'ontologically secure.' This is to suggest that vision loss calls into question people's sense of their inner consistency, substantiality, and worth. It forces them to wonder if they are indeed real, alive, and whole. They must question themselves as 'real' because they focus inordinately upon their otherwise taken-for-granted lives. The recipes by which they judged 'Who am I?' have, at best, been placed in doubt. They must question themselves as 'alive' because their anchors in the world, their bodies, can no longer easily access the physical and social worlds and their hold on space and time are so apparently altered. They must question themselves as 'whole' because the relationship between consciousness (goals, plans, purposes) and their physical and social environments has been obscured. With the future so questionable, the present so demanding, and the past beset by inappropriate recipes and recollections, visually-impaired older persons often find it difficult to realize their intentions for the world. Uncertain intentions are compounded by equally uncertain physical and social environments. Because new visually-impaired older persons question their sense of themselves as real, alive, and whole, ontological insecurity lurks in the problematics of their day-to-day lives.

For people who experienced new vision loss along with the other losses or discontinuities of old age, later life was shown to be characterized by polar outcomes to the challenges posed to their ontological security – integrity versus despair. The task for newly visually-impaired older persons is to discover continuity where none is readily apparent, to define their situation in terms which make it acceptable, and to come to grips with their character as still active, alive, and whole. As observed earlier, this is the essential problem of age identity-in-the-world. While some people vacillated between potential outcomes, for those who accomplished these tasks, old age was characterized by integrity: for those who failed to do so, later life left them to their own despair.

It is only for those people who end up despairing about their lot in life that age-related vision loss can be metaphorically represented by the title of this book – *Day Brought Back My Night*. And even for these people, the 'darkness' of night does not represent their experience of vision loss *per se*. The physiological condition of 'blindness' (a relative term in its own right, given that the defining of visual acuity has a certain 'constructed' quality about it) is seldom experienced as darkness. Most people, especially those who experience vision loss in late life, will have remaining vision which includes light perception. Yet those who despair do experience blindness as 'darkness'. But here we mean the 'darkness' of ontological insecurity, the 'darkness' of living a life that doesn't make sense. Even those people who end up achieving integrity know something of darkness in these terms. As we have seen, people universally experienced a sort of disorientation, a sort of ontological 'vertigo,' when they first learned that they were losing their sight. As such, all people who go through the loss of sight know something about the feelings of people who eventually end up in despair. The difference, of course, lies in their eventual discovery that they could remain active (not just in the sense of 'keeping busy' but also in the sense of remaining an 'actor' in the full sense of that word) and remain a full participant in the world. For those people who achieve integrity, who achieve ontological security, 'darkness' is inappropriate as a way of describing their physical circumstance and it is even metaphorically inappropriate for describing their hold on the world. For them, the world makes sense, there isn't any ontological vertigo (at least no more than for the next person).

The struggle to achieve ontological security, that is integrity, rests largely in the people's ability to transcend their individuality. For those visually-impaired older persons who come to terms with the problematics of their sensory decline, there was a characteristic transcending of their own problems, their own pain, their own fears. Some transcended the failings of their bodies through the sacred legitimation of commonsense theodicies. Some transcended the problematics of their present through the discovery of attitudinal continuity between the triumphs and disappointments of past, present, and future. Some transcended their daily difficulties by identifying with all those who shared in their vision loss (predecessors, contemporaries, heirs). Still others transcended the loss of their previous social contacts by searching out new social arrangements with which they could affiliate and whose goals, purposes, and aims they could adopt. Common to all 'roads to integrity' was the ability of visually-impaired older persons actively to restore the intentional unity of their lives, their projects, their relevances in relation to their changing bodily experience and shifting social environment. In this way, persons who achieved integrity (and hence remained ontologically secure) came to view their suffering, their limitations, their misfortune, as encompassed by some greater whole (the whole of the life course, the whole of fellow blind persons, or the whole of some sacred agenda).

The essential problem of identity-in-the-world, then, is satisfied when the individual arrives at (or returns to) an ontologically secure sense of her/his continuity, situation, and character in spite of the apparent discontinuities, challenges, and problematics which may present themselves. By and large, this ontologically secure sense of continuity, situation, and character is achieved when the interrelated components of identity-in-the-world – that is, consciousness, bodily experience, and social world – are made to jive or fit with one another. In the face of disruption to any one of these components, this jive or fit is achieved when individuals restore their unity through some sort of experiential overview, some greater whole, that transcends any one aspect of identity-in-the-world which may, for the moment, be brought into relief.

Conceiving identity, aging, and vision loss

If there is one insight into human experience with which this study seems to resonate, it is the notion that our lives must be imbued with meaning. The central feature of human experience, in other words – pervading the stories of people's confrontation with the loss of sight – is people's ongoing struggle to achieve some meaningful ordering of the physical and social environments within which they find themselves enwebbed. Once again, as Berger *et al.* (1973) have suggested, this is precisely what it means to be 'human' in the first place. Being 'human' is actively to provide order to one's 'reality' and 'to give sense to the business of living.'

Our attempts to 'give sense to the business of living' extend to all aspects of our lives. We must, for example, make sense of the world that we experience as outside ourselves. We do this for very pragmatic reasons. We desire that the world at least appears knowable and predictable. In order for this to be possible, we order the world into meaningful categories – humans from non-humans, animals from insects, animate creatures from inanimate objects, etc.

Just as we need to make sense of the world that surrounds us, we need to make sense of our place in that world. We bestow meaning upon our relationships to objects: I know this is my book not yours; I know that I can use this chair to sit on if I'm tired and yet I can use it to stand on if I need to reach something outside my grasp. We bestow meaning upon our relationships to other people: I can speak to others by virtue of the order imposed by rules of grammar and shared vocabulary; I know what behavior suits one interactive situation and not another; I know which person is a friend and which is a foe. We even bestow meaning upon our relationship to society and its institutions, as well as to the sacred cosmos.

We are assisted in this meaning-giving activity through what Alfred Schutz (1971) has termed 'recipes' or 'typifications.' 'Recipes' are precisely those cognitive categories that allow us to place things, settings, and/or other people in a meaningful way. As

Schutz pointed out, this meaning is not inherent in nature but rather results from our selective or interpretive activity within nature. This, of course, accords an active role to human consciousness in the process through which the world is 'made' or 'constructed.' But, as Schutz also observed, the world is not entirely of our own making. Quite the contrary, our attempts to provide meaning for the world around us are undeniably tied to both our social world (which supplies many of our own cognitive categories) and our bodies (which provide us access to the world around us, as well as act as interpretive yardsticks for judging our relationships to things and others).

Identity, above all else, is also part of this effort to give sense to the business of living. It is the person's attempt meaningfully to order her/his own situation, continuity, and character. Identity is not, however, an ethereal process. On the contrary, people's attempts to understand themselves and their world as they go through the loss of sight demonstrates that identity formation and maintenance are distinctively 'intentional' processes. This is to say that people's attempts to order their situation, continuity, and character always take place in relation to (and are facilitated by) the physical and social environments, in view of which their situation, continuity, and character make sense in the first place. As the phenomenological dictum suggests, 'people exist for the world and the world exists for people.' In other words, identity has a referent quality. While it necessarily addresses a subjective process, it also refers to the objective world (both physical and social) which surrounds the individual and informs her/his perceptions of her/himself. This is, of course, the importance of the phenomenological use of hyphenated expressions. 'Identity' becomes 'identity-in-the-world.' This is to suggest that one's self-appraisals of situation, continuity, and character are inseparable from and refer to the objective world in which such appraisals occur.

Correspondingly, as we have seen, identity-in-the-world must be conceived in terms of two ongoing dialectics which, in turn, are also bound to one another. The first of them can be described as an 'internal dialectic' between individual consciousness and bodily experience. Because the body accompanies people throughout their involvement in the world, provides them with a sense of time and space, and mediates their actions in and upon their environment, it is ludicrous to speak of consciousness (especially as it appraises situation, continuity, and character) apart from bodily experience. The second dialectic can be described as 'external' and refers to the relationship between consciousness and the social

119

world. Because one's self appraisals take place in and are maintained by interaction with others and because the very vocabulary of self-expressions is provided in a shared social context, it is equally unhelpful to speak of consciousness apart from one's involvement in the world with others.

Yet bodily and/ or social experiences are devoid of human meaning apart from the subject's active struggle to make them meaningful in view of her/ his own set of personal goals, commitments, relevances, and purposes. Consciousness, bodily experience, and social world are thus inextricably bound to one another, and to lose any one of them is to lose the 'whole' of identity-in-the-world.

Identity-in-the-world must simultaneously account for embodied experience, spatiality (the 'here' supplied by the body anchored in the world), temporality (the experience of the 'now' juxtaposed between past and future), and interrelations with other people, ranging from the mechanics of interaction to commitments with others in organizational contexts. All of these elements of identity-in-the-world implicate the aging process. To speak of the present is to speak of a person located somewhere within the lifelong process of growing up and growing old. To speak of space is to speak of one's locations among objects (physical and social) as mediated by an aging body. To speak of one's involvement in a shared social environment is to speak of varied propensities toward interaction itself and different opportunities to sustain organizational involvements over the life course. An adequate theory of identity, then, is already a theory of aging.

We are all aging and our physiological location between birth and death is indisputably a defining quality of that process. Although we might wish otherwise at times, our bodies will age and we will die. Nevertheless, our knowledge of what it means to age and our estimation of our own location within the aging process is not a matter of physiology: it is a matter of our own conscious attempts to make sense of ourselves and our relationship to the world. This is the primary difference between human and non-human aging. Certainly animals go through a maturational process that is in many ways similar to humans. But animals do not 'know' what it means to age and grow old.

Furthermore, our own conscious attempts to make sense of ourselves in terms of the aging process implicate the social world. Humans may come to 'know' themselves as child, adolescent, young adult, middle aged, or old. But it is society that provides us with the lines of demarcation that separate childhood from adolescence, adolescence from young adulthood, young adulthood from middle age, middle age from old age, and the like.

Furthermore, every so often society will decide to change these lines of demarcation, and these changes have to be understood in terms of changing social conditions, not just shifting personal priorities. The social historical era within which a person lives will offer up varied opportunities to her/him. These varied opportunities likely lead to varied self-appraisals. As David Hackett Fischer (1978) has argued, to know old age in colonial America, for example, was to know 'veneration' (a sort of combination of respect and worship). Certainly this provided a sort of social backdrop for knowing what it meant to grow old that is quite different from the social backdrop provided in the United States of the late twentieth century and against which today's older people make sense of their lives. Finally, the technological and economic accomplishments of a given society (in a given age or in a given part of the world) will help define the parameters of the life course itself – influencing longevity as well as survival rates. The social world, in other words, provides a context within which our physiological aging as well as our projects, plans, and self-estimations occur. We must stop short of assuming, however, that our estimations of aging are socially determined. We must also remind ourselves that the interplay between self, body, and social world – that is part of the aging process – is not bound to one historical period or to one social location.

Like identity and aging, vision loss must also be conceived of in terms of the interplay of self, body, and social world. One cannot act as if the loss of sight makes no difference to the people who experience it. Vision loss owes to one or another physiological change in the eye. It forces people to rely more on tactile information than they would if they retained their sight. It removes distant visual cues from that information that is readily available for judging their place among objects and other people. Like the physiological aging of our bodies, vision loss is a defining quality of the phenomenon we term 'blindness' or 'severe vision loss.' Like age-related changes in the body, vision loss cannot be wished away.

Nevertheless (and, here again, vision loss is like the physiological component of aging) the physiological changes in the eye that help to define blindness or severe vision loss tell us very little about what it means to be blind or to be severely visually impaired. Just as an animal cannot 'know' what it means to grow old, an animal cannot 'know' what it means to lose sight. A person experiencing vision loss is left to make sense of just what vision loss will mean to her/him, why she/he (and not someone else) experienced it and if she/he is a different person because of it.

A person's attempts to give sense to the business of being blind or the business of being severely visually impaired will also take place against a social backdrop. As Michael Monbeck (1973) has carefully documented, the western world's present-day attitudes toward blindness have emerged from the literature of ancient times, mythological tales, and religious scripture and teachings. This observation is not only important to understanding the experience of blindness in the past. Such sources have shaped the 'stigma' which has been socially attached to the physiological phenomenon we term blindness. Helplessness, misery, and self-pity are no more intrinsic to the loss of sight than is aesthetic giftedness, increased powers of concentration, or imagination. They are, however, part of the types or recipes possessed by the social audience that any person experiencing vision loss will confront. Such attitudes may close some doors and open others in terms of opportunities that are cut off or made available. This is why Erving Goffman (1963) said we really need a language of relationships not attributes to understand what stigma (of all sorts) is about. Yet social determinism must again be rejected, for, despite the negative stereotypes that surround blindness, to experience vision loss is not to end up being helpless, miserable, reduced to self-pity, aesthetically gifted, or blessed with superior imagination. To experience vision loss is to confront a social audience that will view the person differently by virtue of her/his physiological loss. Yet the person experiencing vision loss, like everyone else, must make a world for themselves in relation to their changing (and changed) bodies and the constraints of the social world. They, like everyone else, will vary in the extent to which they can make the business of living seem sensible.

Generalizing beyond aging and vision loss

There seems to be little doubt that new vision loss accompanying advancing age prompts dramatic changes in the individual's personal agenda, relationships with physical objects, and her/his interaction with other people. There is equally little doubt that, as such, new vision loss among older people explodes the taken-for-granted nature of their identity-in-the-world, thus revealing the intricacies of its dialectical components. One might reasonably ask, however, are there limitations which must be imposed upon attempts to generalize the observations of this study beyond its specific empirical focus?

New vision loss certainly represents an amplified instance of the manifestations of physical decline which confront all persons in the later years of life. One obvious question, then, is to what degree are the experiences of newly visually-impaired persons unique? It is quite clear that the majority of older persons will never experience severe (newsprint disability) impairment of their sight as did the respondents in this study. As such, some of the discontinuities experienced by the people here would not be salient to most older people. Yet a surprisingly large portion of the older population is affected by some sort of chronic condition. As Robert Atchley (1985: 74) has noted, less than 15 per cent of persons over age 65 have no chronic conditions. About one-half of all persons over age 65 have two or more. Chronic conditions, as defined by the National Center for Health Statistics (NCHS), include various impairments (vision loss, hearing loss, speech defects, paralysis, absence of extremities, impairment of extremities) and chronic diseases (arthritis, rheumatism, heart conditions, high blood pressure, diabetes, chronic bronchitis, etc.). With few exceptions, the prevalence of chronic conditions steadily increases in older age groups. Each of these chronic conditions carries with it a host of daily problematics. Loss of hearing (the most frequently experienced impairment in older persons), for example, carries with it as many if not more problems than does vision loss (see Oyer and Oyer 1976; also see Gaylene Becker's examination of the aged deaf 1980). Chronic diseases can surpass vision impairment in their limiting impact upon people's activities (as is the case, most notably, with heart conditions, arthritis, and rheumatism – all of which surpass vision impairment as causes of limitation to activity (see Atchley 1985)). In all, 39 per cent of persons over age 65, with some chronic condition, report that they have a resulting limitation to some major activity. In other words, each chronic condition, in its own right, calls into question the limited nature of a person's duration in the world.

Vision loss does carry with it some unique personally-, physically-, and socially-imposed limitations to activity, as well as specific contacts with service providers, but it is nevertheless representative of that greater whole of physical and social challenges which beset people as they approach later life. Many persons are similarly reminded of their inevitable biological decline by the host of other impairments and chronic diseases spoken of above. Each of these conditions also carry with them limitations to activity, intense and extended contact with service and medical professionals, feelings of fear, disbelief, panic, etc., and can be equally or even more socially isolating (as in the case of deafness). Still other persons are reminded (although admittedly less dramatically) of their limited duration by the signs of aging shared universally by people growing up and growing old. Loss of body weight, skin and pigment alterations, slowing reaction time, decreasing muscular strength, and other visible changes of the human organism become apparent to all people in later life. Older persons also universally experience the loss of friends and family through institutionalization, illness, and death, which was addressed earlier. In other words, while to greater and lesser extents, all older people experience the discontinuities of the aging process and as such all must face the problem of age identity-in-the-world.

Age-identity-in-the-world: a lifelong process

Beyond the similar experiences of people facing discontinuities in later life, the problem of age identity-in-the-world (that is, coming to terms with one's situation, continuity, and character in view of personal projects in relation to a physical and social context) faces people throughout the life course. The problem of age identity-in-the-world is by no means unique either to old age or to any one of its accompanying physical or social changes. New vision loss and/or old age only bring into relief the dynamics which are at play for everyone, regardless of age or physical condition. Subjective reality is precarious throughout the process of growing up and growing old. 'Human existence is an ongoing "balancing act" between man and his body and man and his world' (Berger 1967: 5–6). Whenever one experiences physical change (from the development of physical prowess in childhood to the decline of the same in old age) or the social world begins to totter (significant others are lost for whatever reason – including geographical or occupational mobility, in addition to institutionalization, illness, and death) or one's personal agenda shifts (a person's judgement regarding her/his situation dictates a different course of action), the individual is reminded that the maintenance of age identity-in-the-world is an ongoing struggle to make its components jive or fit. As Erikson observes, identity 'is never gained nor maintained once and for all. Like a good conscience it is constantly lost and regained' (quoted in Strauss 1969: 109). Sharon Kaufman has, more recently, taken this position as well, insisting that 'identity is created and recreated over time as a person progresses through the life span' (1986: 151).

Here again, let us return to the theme of narrative that was taken up earlier in Chapter 4. It was suggested that people find order in their lives through the telling and retelling of their lives through personal narratives. Such 'world making' is not limited to later life (whether or not one accepts the notion that life review is more important here than at other stages of the life course). Quite the contrary, the narrative or world-making process accompanies every turn of human experience. Jean-Paul Sartre insists that the stories we tell to ourselves and to others about our lives take otherwise disconnected events, characteristics, situations, and put them into some sort of meaningful order. As the protagonist Roquentin in *Nausea* (a novel that explores this issue of narrative as world making) observes, the 'adventure' of living comes from the 'way in which the moments are linked together.' But collecting (or better *re*collecting) various aspects of our lives into some meaningful order – an order bestowed from the present with its own set of interpretive priorities – is part of childhood, adolescence, middle adulthood, as well as old age. At any age, people must conjure up some meaning for their world and their experience in it. This gives people a sense of both personal power (the power to create 'adventures' out of our past) and personal responsibility (the responsibility for things that did or did not 'work out'). World making, in these terms, may even take on the qualities of 'magic.' 'There is a kind of magic in recollection, a magic that one feels at every age' (de Beauvoir 1972: 361).

Ernest Becker has pointed out that this sense of recollecting or world creating may, at times, make us feel more like gods than magicians.

> Man has a symbolic identity that brings him sharply out of nature. He is a symbolic self, a creature with a name, a life history. He is a creator with a mind that soars out to speculate about atoms and infinity, who can place himself imaginatively at a point in space and contemplate bemusedly his own planet. This immense expansion, this dexterity, this ethereality, this self-consciousness gives to man literally the status of a small god in nature, as the Renaissance thinkers knew. (Becker 1973: 26)

But Becker also observes that this seemingly ethereal quality of the process of world creating gives way to the realization that we are inescapably tied to our bodies – bodies that age, bodies that eventually die.

> Yet at the same time, as the Eastern sages also knew, man is a worm and food for worms. This is the paradox: he is out of nature and hopelessly in it; he is dual, up in the stars and yet housed in a heart-pumping, breath-gasping body . . . .. His body is a material fleshy casing that is alien to him in many ways – the

strangest and most repugnant way being that it aches and bleeds and will decay and die. (Becker 1973: 26)

According to Becker, all this means that we face an 'existential paradox,' the condition of 'individuality within finitude,' choice and creative capacities within constraints imposed by our very physical being. We might hasten to add here that the existential paradox is not contained in old age: it is contained in our very humanness.

To put Becker's point in language that we have already developed here, we are 'bound' to our bodies. A person is not determined by her/his body nor the changes that body goes through during the life course. The individual is, none the less, bound to it. This is one lesson that the experience of aging and new vision loss has to offer. We cannot deny (experientially nor in our attempts to understand human experience theoretically) that ours is, as the phenomenologists call it, 'embodied' existence. We play out our lives, we realize our goals in our bodies – bodies that are subject to change.

Another lesson is that our boundedness does not end here. We are also 'bound' to the social context within which we find ourselves. As was observed at the close of Chapter 4, a person's recollections of her/his past and the narrative she/he tells about it depends upon a plausibility structure or social base that will support the recollection or narrative as 'plausible' and 'real.' Again, our world making or creating is not determined by the social context any more than it is determined by our bodies. But our world making or creating is no more ethereal in the sense of being free from the social system of determination than it is ethereal in the sense of being free from physical existence. Such is the limited nature of human freedom.

A final lesson must be gleaned from our exploration of new vision loss among older persons. That lesson is that we all face the challenge of balancing these three components of age-identity-in-the-world and as such we all struggle to maintain ontological insecurity. The struggle to achieve ontological security, to maintain a sense of ourselves as continuous, alive, and whole, is not a problem of any one age. Alternatively put, ontological insecurity is something that can confront any one of us, at any age. This means that integrity (conceived of as the successful balancing of the components of identity-in-the-world) and despair (when the balancing act fails) are polar outcomes of any age. There is little doubt that older people must struggle between integrity and despair, must struggle with ontological security/insecurity. But then, so too must we all. Day could bring back the night for any one of us, at any age, should we lose the precarious balance of identity-in-the-world.

Changing bodies, changing social circumstances, must be confronted in people's ongoing attempts to render their lives both meaningful and in some way unified. This is, for one last time, precisely the problem of age-identity-in-the-world. At the risk of being even more redundant, not one of these aspects of age-identity-in-the-world can be understood without considering the other two, nor is the task of balancing them located in any one moment of the lifelong aging process. Thus the problem of age-identity-in-the-world is faced by everyone, regardless of their location in that lifelong process of growing up and growing old. It is, perhaps, more easily scrutinized in those moments when its taken-for-granted nature has been exploded. The agenda for further research into age-identity-in-the-world must necessarily include and should set as a high priority the investigation of the interplay of self, body, and social world at varying points throughout the aging process and in the face of different disruptions which might reveal their complexity. Various biological disruptions at different points in the aging process beg to be examined. Of equal interest, however, would be the scrutiny of age-identity-in-the-world as it is disrupted by explosions of other of its various components – acute disruptions to the person's social world or personal agenda. In any case one would expect to ask the essential question regarding age-identity-in-the-world: How does one retain an ontologically secure sense of situation, continuity, and character in the face of an ever-changing biological organism, shifting social world, or an active consciousness whose goals, plans, and relevances are susceptible to modification? As in the case of age-related vision loss, the answers that we find to these questions will tell us a great deal about the essential human drama in which we are all key players.

Appendix one

Methods of procedure

In part due to the sparse nature of research on older visually-impaired persons and in part due to the theoretical orientation employed in this study, it is particularly important that the integrity of the loss of sight in late life be preserved. This was accomplished by selecting a research strategy that concentrated on actors' own experiences – that is, their priorities, their plans, their hopes, and their fears. Who, after all, is really in a better place to tell us something about what it means to lose one's sight? True, older visually-impaired persons are not in a position to tell us much about the demographic trends that we can anticipate for blindness in the year 2000, but they are the only people who can tell us what it means to go through the loss.

Psathas (1968) has suggested that one of the most effective means by which the integrity of the social actor's own experience can be preserved is through the use of 'cooperative procedures.' This refers specifically to attempts to elicit a cooperative dialogue with the social actor. This is, of course, partially the intent of participant observation – commonly associated with and utilized by symbolic and phenomenological inter-actionists (see Bogdan and Taylor 1975). Yet one of the most fruitful of cooperative procedures, though in recent years under-utilized, is the life-history method (see Angell 1945; Becker 1966; Young 1966; and Faraday and Plummer 1979 for extensive reviews of the research in this tradition). As Becker describes it, the life-history method is most concerned with precisely the 'faithful rendering of the subject's experiences and interpret-ations of the world he lives in' (1966: vi). It is the life-history method that is employed here. More specifically, it could be termed 'multi-subject topical life history' (see Denzin 1970) inasmuch as it concentrates on one phase of subjects' lives (that surrounding the loss of sight) and approaches multiple respondents in like circumstance instead of only one informant.

The chief advantages of this approach are three-fold according to Faraday and Plummer (1979). In the first place, its overt goal is to establish 'reality' as it appears to the subject rather than as it appears to the social scientific observer. Second, it allows the observer to focus upon the processual character of everyday experience. Rather than imposing an order or form upon the world of everyday life which may be inappropriate, the life history aims at allowing the order imposed by the social actors to surface while also leaving room for the ambiguity, confusion, and contradictions which are also part of subjective experience. Third, the life-history approach focuses on the 'totality' of human experience. By maximizing the opportunity for the actor to tell her/his story in her/his own terms, the observer is forced to confront the full complexity of the subject's involvement in the world. It becomes more difficult, in other words, for the social scientist to 'amputate' a unitary aspect of what is, from the subject's point of view, a much more complex phenomenon. For these reasons the life-history method is particularly well suited to the exploratory goals of the study and allows elderly people to tell their own stories.

During the fall and winter of 1979–80, twenty persons were interviewed regarding their experience of vision loss. I used what Richardson (1965: 45) has called the 'non-schedule standardized interview' format. This is to say that while similar classes of information were asked of each respondent, both the specific way in which the questions were posed and the sequence in which they were asked varied somewhat from subject to subject. This allowed me to tailor the interview to what was known about the subject's background (such factors as extent and chronology of visual impairment) and to their personal priorities which became clear during the course of the interview.

From the standpoint of some life-history proponents, the use of the non-schedule standardized-interview format moves the personal document away from the subject's 'pure' account on the 'continuum of contamination' (see Faraday and Plummer 1979: 787). By comparison, self-written autobiographies and diaries are relatively unfettered in their ability to offer purely subjective accounts of individual experience. The introduction of even the broadest parameters of researcher interests may be judged to contaminate the personal nature of the resulting data. This concern had to be balanced, however, against the need to guide the subject to the topics which were judged relevant to the experience of vision loss (see Denzin 1970; Bogdan and Taylor 1975).

To minimize the dangers of contamination of the subjects' personal accounts, painstaking pretest procedures become critical to the life-history method. It is essential that the classes of information and rough outline of questions to be asked in the non-schedule standardized interview are formulated in a cooperative dialogue with similarly-situated people as those upon whom the research focuses. Correspondingly, prior to interviewing the twenty persons whose stories are found in this study, I talked extensively with other elderly persons who were blind or visually impaired and established 'overlapping relevances' (Cicourel 1964: 79). Rather than testing specific predefined questions, I generated a life-history interview schedule through 'systematic thematic analysis.' As Faraday and Plummer describe this process, through a slow and yet methodical interchange between observer and subjects,

> there comes a point when the subject is more or less allowed to speak for him or herself but where the sociologist slowly accumulates a series

of themes – partly derived from the subject's account but partly derived from sociological theory. (Faraday and Plummer 1979: 787)

The life-history interviews covered a number of key topical areas – biographical information, experience of vision loss (chronology, extent of impairment, limitations imposed by vision loss, and other problems incurred), sense of bodily well-being, reflections on bodily changes since the advent of vision loss, relationships with others (both significant and less significant others), goals, fears, concerns, and various other aspects of the person's view of her/himself.

In an effort to preserve rapport during the interview sessions and not overly to tire either interviewee or interviewer, two sessions lasting approximately two hours each were scheduled with all twenty subjects. With many of the people more time was required and an additional session was scheduled after the second meeting. The interviews were conducted at their convenience and in their homes. Such considerations seemed necessary investments for the research. The topics covered often brought back painful recollections and the comfort of the home, as well as some minimal personal commitment from the interviewer, were essential prerequisites.

The intensive interviews took place in the middle of a year-and-a-half period, during which an attempt was made to understand more fully not only the world of those experiencing blindness and visual impairment but also the world of those who provide services to them. Both groups have their respective reasons for viewing sociologists (or researchers more generally) with some suspicion, and yet, in time, I was able to minimize these suspicions and to allay some of their fears. I attended meetings of the Lion's Club and local blind consumer groups, Christmas parties hosted by the latter, workshops on blindness at the American Foundation for the Blind in New York City, and planning sessions of both state and local-level service providers. I was invited into the homes of individuals who were blind and professionals alike, and befriended by both. These contacts fulfilled the role of the informant critical to all qualitative work and also made the research activity all the more urgent to me.

Contextualizing the life-history informants

In doing life-history research, one must show some caution so as not to overstate the representativeness of her/his single case or even multiple cases (as used in this study). Ernest Burgess was acutely aware of this issue, as is evidenced in his discussion of Shaw's study of delinquency in *The Jack Roller* (1966: 184ff.). Burgess warned that Shaw's life history of the single case of Stanley did not exhaust the phenomenon of juvenile delinquency (not even for Chicago, where Stanley resided). He argued 'no single case could be representative of all the many variations of personality, of the permutations of situations and the diversity of experiences' (1966: 184). Nevertheless, Burgess suggested that even single cases are 'typical' to a certain degree. As he again observed of Shaw's study of Stanley,

Appendix 1

The case of Stanley appears also to be typical in a more real sense than can be verified by any statistical calculation. It is typical (i.e. belonging to the type) in the same way that every case is a representation of its kind or species. . . . It may not be the best specimen, perhaps only a good specimen or even a poor specimen. There can be no doubt that any case, good, bad or indifferent, is a specimen of the species to which it belongs. (Burgess 1966: 185–6)

Thus every single case of new vision loss is, in some sense, 'typical' of the phenomenon, even though it may only be a good, poor, or indifferent instance of the same.

It is, however, possible to improve upon the degree to which the researcher can protect against the peculiarities of her/his case(s). Burgess noted, 'in analyzing any case as a specimen of the other cases of its kind, it is desirable and perhaps necessary always to make comparisons with other cases, both those which are like and unlike it' (1966: 187). Similarly, Denzin (1970: 221) suggests that it is always useful for the life-history observer to 'place his subjects within the total range of units his single case represents.' He goes on to argue,

If the life history is of a juvenile delinquent, for instance, then a demographic and ecological analysis of the population of delinquents from which the single case is drawn must be presented. This permits generalizations to the broader population by studying a subunit from it – a basic principle of statistical sampling theory. (Denzin 1970: 221)

This study avoids some of the difficulties of one-case analysis by using a multi-subject sample (see Bogdan and Taylor 1975: 118). Beyond this, statements about the broader population of visually-impaired older persons can be enhanced by presenting demographic characteristics of the life-history informants so that comparisons with the 'total range of units' can be made.

Table A1.1 Age distribution of the life-history informants

Age group	Number of respondents
55–9	3
60–4	4
65–9	3
70–4	2
75–9	2
80+	6
Total	20

The age distribution of the life-history informants (at the time of the interview) appears in Table A1.1. Not surprisingly, 40 per cent of the life-history sample were 75 years of age or older. This seems to correspond with the general trend (suggested by the National Center for Health Statistics 'Health Interview Survey' and reported in Chapter 1) associated with age and severe visual impairment.

Table A1.2   Gender composition of the life-history informants

Gender	Life-history sample (%)
Male	35
Female	65
Total	100

In considering the gender composition of the informants in this study, the national population of persons with severe visual impairments is again approximated. Of the informants, 35 per cent (seven) were male and 65 per cent (thirteen) were female. While the data are not directly comparable (i.e. NCHS data are presented only for persons 65 years of age or older, as opposed to the age 55 and older used in the life-history sample), the similarities are striking. For the national population of severely visually-impaired persons, the gender distribution is 34.5 per cent males and 65.5 per cent females. Given the general (sex ratio) tendency for there to be fewer males than females with increasing age (for a general discussion of this tendency see Atchley 1985), the differences in age criteria used in presenting the gender composition of the life-history informants and the US population of severely visually-impaired persons probably mean that males are slightly under-represented among the life-history informants. This speculation is supported by looking at the gender composition of the 1979 US population over age 55.

Table A1.3   Household incomes of the life-history informants

Income	Life-history informants (%)
$10,000 or more	22.2
$5,000–9,999	27.8
$5,000 or less	50.0
Total	100.0
	(N=18)

Similarly, the income levels reported by life-history informants and those for the US population of severely visually-impaired persons approximated one another (income data of national population of severely visually-impaired persons has been summarized by Kirchner and Peterson 1979); 22.2 per cent (compared to 18.8 per cent of severely visually-impaired persons 65 and older) had incomes of more than

$10,000, 27.8 per cent (compared to 25.4 per cent) had incomes between $5,000 and $9,999, and 50 per cent (compared to 55.8 per cent) had incomes of less than $5,000. Differences between these two groups may well be a function of inflation between 1977 (when NCHS figures were released) and 1979 (when first contacts with informants were made).

Table A1.4 Years of school completed for the life-history informants

Years of school completed	Life-history informants (%)
Elementary (1–8 years)	30
High school (1–4 years)	60
College (1 or more years)	10
Total	100

Some comparisons can also be made between the life-history informants and the US population of persons over age 55 with regard to educational background. Table A1.4 indicates the educational background of the life-history informants which are similar (in most cases) to the national population of persons 55 and older. In 1977, for example, 44.5 per cent of persons 55 and older had at least some high-school education, compared to 40 per cent of the life-history informants (US Census 1978). Only two (10 per cent) informants had, however, any college experience, as compared to 18 per cent of persons 55 or older in 1977 (US Census 1978). This suggests that college-educated persons are likely under-represented among the life-history informants.

Table A1.5 Living arrangements of the life-history informants

Living arrangements	Life-history informants (%)
Alone	45
With spouse	40
With family	10
With friends	5
Total	100

The majority of the life-history informants either lived alone or with their spouses (see Table A1.5). This is also true for older persons as a whole. As Treas (1975: 94) has observed in her studies of the elderly, it would seem 'most older people have chosen to live apart, that is alone or with their spouse.' They do not, by and large, live with family or friends. This is certainly evident in the life-history informants. One noteworthy difference is, however, that a higher proportion of the life-history informants live alone when compared with other older persons (the

Census Bureau reported that in 1975 14.8 per cent of males and 37.3 per cent of females over age 65 were living alone).

Table A1.6   Major causes of vision loss in the life-history sample

Cause of vision loss	Number of respondents
Macular degeneration	7
Cataracts	4
Glaucoma	3
Diabetic retinopathy	2
Retinitis pigmentosa	2
Retinal detachment	1
Vascular occlusions	1
Total	20

There are several other characteristics of the life-history informants that deserve attention. In Chapter 1, various etiologies of vision loss were discussed at considerable length. All of the major forms of vision loss reported in that discussion were evidenced in the life-history informants (as shown in Table A1.6). Comparisons with a national population are virtually meaningless as so many cases of severe vision loss go unreported and inasmuch as a professional diagnosis is required (which makes the NCHS data problematic for comparison purposes here).

Table A1.7   Years since 'vision loss caused major difficulties with everyday life' for life-history informants

Years since onset	Number of life-history informants
1–2	4
3–4	3
5–6	4
7–8	3
9–10	6
Total	20

Lastly, as suggested earlier, a delimiting criterion of years passed since onset of vision difficulties was used to select people for the pool of life-history informants. Informants were evenly dispersed along this variable, with the exception of those first experiencing their vision difficulties nine to ten years earlier (with more informants falling into this category than the others, ranging from one to eight years since onset).

These background characteristics of the life-history informants should help place the participants in this study in some general relationship with the overall population of elderly, as well as the national population of persons experiencing severe visual loss. They don't, of course, insure that informants' responses are entirely representative of the 'type,' that is of all persons who experience the loss of sight in late life. They do, however, reassure us that they are not fundamentally at odds with the 'type.'

Appendix two

Rethinking traditional theories of identity, aging, and vision loss

I would like to consider here the inadequacies of theories of identity, aging, and vision loss that do not simultaneously account for the actor making choices about her/his life within the contexts (systems of determination) of bodily and social experience. I have avoided placing this discussion within the text so as not to burden those readers who may not be familiar with, and who have little interest in, traditional approaches within the social sciences to these problem areas. I consider the implications to be important, and my placing of this discussion in an appendix should not be construed as 'relegating' this consideration to a place of secondary importance. I would also caution that this section is not intended to be a comprehensive 'literature review.' Rather, I have attempted to pick representatives of the various approaches to identity, aging, and vision loss that have 'lost' one or another of the component parts I consider essential to understanding each of these phenomena.

My argument for 'identity-in-the-world' – conceived of as people's ongoing struggle to make sense of their situation, continuity, and character – carries with it a necessary criticism of those previous approaches to the problem of identity which forfeit the full complexity of individuals' relationships to the world around them (see Ainlay and Redfoot 1982 for a thorough critique). As I will suggest, this does not mean that previous theories of identity have nothing to say to us about how the balancing of self, body, and social world is managed. It means that they have either:

1 not recognized that all these component parts need be accounted for; or
2 they have tried to lend a sort of causal superiority (or primacy) to one or another of the component parts.

Approaches informed largely by Meadean social psychology have tended, for example, to adopt a sort of 'social behaviorism' that was advocated by George Herbert Mead himself. Describing the dynamics of the 'construction' of consciousness becomes Mead's major concern in his *Mind, Self and Society* (1934). Therein, he describes the 'genesis of the self' (see especially 1934: 144ff.). This 'genesis' is indicative of the causal priority which he ascribes to the social. He insists that the infant is not born with a self but rather develops it through interaction with the social environment. At first this occurs through the imitative process of 'taking the role' of specific others. Children 'play at' being a parent, for example (1934: 150). They do so by reenacting the stimuli (i.e. gestures) which have been observed in the person they are imitating and which have called out certain responses in themselves. In such a way the initial basis for understanding other role players is established. The further development of the self is enhanced when the child begins to participate in 'games' (1934: 151). Mead distinguishes the game stage in that it depends upon rules and a number of participants. These factors force the child to take into account the roles and attitudes of multiple others involved in the game (1934: 153–4). This game stage is only the gateway to the culmination of the genesis of the self, i.e. the mature social self is that which is able to treat itself as object. This is the stage at which Mead argues the child takes on the attitude of the 'generalized other' (1934: 154). Rather than governing her/his action in terms of specific others, the child now governs actions in terms of more abstract principles and norms of the larger social community. In this way, Mead argues, the individual now has a unified vantage point from which to experience her/himself as a unified object.

This review of Mead's discussion of the genesis of the self is not aimed at demonstrating the ludicrousness of his analysis. On the contrary, Mead's discussion of the interplay of society and consciousness is perhaps the most adequate penetration of this one aspect of the subjective experience of oneself. Mead's error is not so much one of commission as one of omission. His criticism of idealism and behaviorism led him to focus on a unidimensional aspect of what we have argued to be the full complexity of identity-in-the-world which necessarily makes the self arising out of social processes just one aspect of a multidimensional problem. Mead's failure was not to recognize this fact. More specifically, he does not allow for an active enough role for the self, nor does he seem to appreciate the central place of the body.

Mead, of course, avoided narrow determinism by discussing the internal dialogue between the 'I' and the 'me' (1934: 173ff.). That part of the self which consists of the attitudes of others organized and taken over by the individual is called the 'me.' However, Mead noted that the self was not exhausted by the 'me.' It also possesses the 'I' which represents the impulsive nature of the individual who is aware of the 'me' and reacts to it. These two moments of the self are important to Mead because they constitute the essentially dialectical nature of human existence which is obtained through socialization (1934: 178). Mead also discussed the ambiguity of situations which force the individual to choose between multiple possible responses (1964: 125–7). His writings in the *Philosophy of the Act* also show a remarkable sensitivity to a more active consciousness (especially in its role in 'impulse' and 'perception' as stages of the 'act') than his writings in *Mind, Self and Society*. This 'promise' in Mead's work has not been fully appreciated by his disciples.

Gregory Stone, for example, believes that the term 'identity' most meaningfully conveys 'what' and 'where' a person is in social terms. Stone insists that 'when one has identity, he is *situated* – that is, cast in the shape of a social object by the acknowledgement of his participation or membership in social relations. One's identity is established when others *place* him as a social object' (1962: 93). Stone sacrifices active consciousness in the constitution of identity by further asserting that identity is an expression of Mead's 'me' (1962: 94). Thus whatever active role consciousness may play in Mead's dialectic of the 'I' and the 'me' is lost in Stone's conception of identity. It is somewhat unfair to single out Stone here. Like Mead himself, we would not want to dismiss Stone's insights. Nevertheless, to lose the active role that individuals play in responding to others' placement of them or to lose the import of the body to people's sense of personal continuity is to lose identity as people experience it in their lives. The desire to lend conceptual simplicity to identity does not merit such a loss.

Another example of problems with previous treatments of identity can be found in the work of Talcott Parsons. To understand the place of identity in Parsons' framework one must begin with his discussion of the 'personality.' The personality is, for Parsons, a partially autonomous system which is interpenetrated by the social, cultural, and behavioral organic systems. Parsons accomplished this theoretical position through a synthesis of the positions of Durkheim and Freud. The plausibility of this synthesis flows from what Parsons sees as the 'convergence' of their views on the importance of the 'internalization of moral norms' (1964: 18ff.). To accomplish this merger Parsons seeks to overcome Freud's failure to treat the interaction of individual personalities as a system and Durkheim's concentration on systems at the expense of interacting personalities (1964: 20).

Parsons promises to develop a view of the personality which emphasizes the relations between that personality and the social system, insisting that

> my view will be that while the main content of the structure of personality is derived from social systems and culture through socialization, the personality becomes an independent system through its own organism and through the uniqueness of its own life experiences: it is not a mere epiphenomenon of the structure of society. (1964: 82)

In spite of his avowal that the personality is an 'independent system,' Parsons doesn't endow the personality with the characteristics and mechanisms by which such independence could be achieved. Rather, he ultimately leaves the reader with what Alfred Baldwin has called the 'impoverishment of the personality' (1961: 186).

Parsons relegates the personality to a position of dependence upon the social, giving the latter logical priority over the former. He concludes that 'not only moral standards but all the components of the common culture are internalized as part of the personality structure' such that 'neither what the human *is* in the most subjective respects, nor what it *means* emotionally, can be understood as given independently of the interactive process itself' (1964: 23). In this light Parsons' concern with socialization processes can be seen as aimed largely at demonstrating how this internalization of 'moral standards' and 'components of common culture' lends to the maintenance of social order (see Parsons 1951, especially Chapter VI).

In his essay on 'The position of identity in the general theory of action' Parsons reaffirms this dependent relationship of the personality to the social system by revealing the former's 'structure' and (directly pertinent to the present interest) the place of identity. Parsons states that 'the structure of the personality as a system is composed of "objects" which have been learned in the course of life experience, that experience having been "codified" in terms of culturally given codes' (1968: 15). It is precisely as a 'structural aspect of the personality of an individual conceived as a system' that Parsons comes to introduce identity. Thus Parsons suggests that identity merely reflects the capacity of the individual to understand her/himself as a social object using socially-supplied codes. In more typical Parsonian terms, identity is the 'pattern-maintenance-code-system' of the individual personality (1968: 20).

It is to Parsons' credit that he denies the separability of organism, individual, and society by insisting 'what is important here is the fundamental insight that the traditional disjunction (which has run so deep in Western Thought) between the organism, the personality of the individual, and the structure of his society and culture is untenable' (1968: 14). To the extent that he describes their 'interpenetration,' Parsons seems to sense (though he never fully grasps) their fundamental interrelatedness. Yet by stressing their systemic independence in his analysis he seems to lose this unity of experience of oneself by attempting to lend the causal priority explicit in his hierarchical arrangement of its components.

Not only does Parsons lose the unity of organism, individual, and society, but, by conceiving these components in systemic and hierarchical terms, he sacrifices any truly active role for consciousness and the importance of the body. By seeing identity as dependent upon the social for both its location in the interactive system and for the very codes by which one interprets the meaning of this location and actions within that system (cognitive and conative aspects) without dealing adequately with its reflexive dimension, Parsons deprives the individual of the active role he at times seeks to provide. He also fails to account adequately, as Dennis Wrong (1970) suggested in his essay 'The oversocialized conception of man in modern sociology,' for people's experience of their bodies.

While it is possible to agree with Wrong that granting logical priority to the social results in an 'oversocialized conception of man' (a criticism which must also extend to Mead and the symbolic interactionists), his embrace of Freud's psychoanalytical approach to the self is untenable. If Mead and Parsons' social priority is not entirely adequate, then neither is the priority which Freud gives to the biological organism.

Freud's theory begins with the 'id,' that web of unconscious impulses that is 'somewhere in direct contrast with somatic processes and takes over from them instinctual needs and gives them mental expression' (Freud 1952: 837). It is the 'psychological underworld' that precedes the more conscious level of the 'ego' and the 'superego' (1952: 830). Or, as Freud elsewhere observes, 'the ego is continued inwards, without any sharp delimitation, into an unconscious mental entity which we designate as the id and for which it serves as a kind of facade' (1961: 13). In Freud's analysis, the id is given both chronological and causal priority. At birth the infant is 'all id' (Erikson 1950: 192). It is in confronting the external world that the 'ego' develops or as Freud put it 'the ego is that part of the id which has been modified by the direct influence of the external world' (1960: 15).

Freud's discussion of the development of the ego in relation to both id and superego is as close as he gets to the notion of identity – which is also Erikson's later point of departure (which will be discussed in a moment). While the development of the ego does not occur in a social vacuum, Freud gives clear priority to the role of the biological instincts, as is evidenced in his discussion of the various stages of development, i.e. 'oral,' 'anal,' and 'genital' (1935: 336–8, and 1953: 135ff. for examples).

Just as Mead's discussion of the 'genesis of the self' proved a useful illustration of the priority he assigned to the social, Freud's discussion of the importance of 'erotogenic zones' demonstrates the priority he lends to biological factors. According to Freud, the early developmental history of the child is best captured by the respective dominance of certain sensitive zones – the oral, the anal, and the genital regions. The child's earliest libidinal pleasures are associated mainly with the mouth. Freud notes that the first object of the oral component of the sexual instinct is the mother's breast which satisfies the infant's need for nutrition (1935: 338, and 1953: 179–80). The child also begins to suck her/his own fingers and uses her/his mouth to explore and test objects of the external world. The child here is primarily 'narcissistic,' deriving most gratification from her/himself and her/his own body, yet she/he begins to learn which actions bring disapproval and as such the differentiation of the ego and id is begun. In a second phase of development the anus becomes the dominant region or erotogenic zone (see 1953: 185ff.). As Benedek observes, 'its double function – retention and elimination – becomes the center of interest and source of pleasure' (1952: 71). In this stage the child must somehow balance the instinctual pleasure of soiling with desire for the mother's approval. Hence toilet training is the first major instance of the ego's struggle for mastery over the id. The third developmental stage is called the genital (or oedipal, phallic, see examples of Freud's discussion 1935: 333ff., and 1953: 187ff.). Where sexual urges in the pre-genital phases were directed toward the child's own body, now they are directed toward the opposite sex parent. Herein one finds the most famous of Freudian concepts – 'penis envy,' 'castration anxiety,' 'oedipal complex,' 'electra complex,' etc. Ultimately, it is during this phase that the structure of the personality becomes more complex and differentiated. The superego develops in conflict with the id and the ego begins to mediate between the two.

The Freudian stage approach to early child development lends to the biological what the Meadian approach attributed to the social. In this way Freud stands in sharp contradistinction to Mead by assigning causal priority to biological factors in development instead of social relationships. By the same token, however, both Freud and Mead propose treatments of the individual as object, battered by internal or external forces.

Perhaps the most recognized author in the Freudian tradition to approach identity is Erik Erikson. Trained in the psychoanalytical tradition, Erikson took on the task of psychosocializing Freud. In his *Childhood and Society* (1950), Erikson built a stage model of individual development which extended Freud's model of infant sexuality. Beginning with Freud's erotogenic categories, Erikson posited that the mind develops progressively through the oral sensory, mascularity-anal, and locomotor-genital stages, in what he called a 'restatement of the theory of infantile sexuality.' He sought to add, however, an accounting of the various social factors which accompany the succession of erotogenic stages. Erikson expanded this discussion of 'infantile sexuality' to other stages and developmental tasks, eight in all, running through the entire life span (his concern with old age or 'maturity' as a psychosocial developmental stage will be discussed more fully later). Erikson's major achievement in his discussion of these developmental stages must be underscored. That is, biosexual development must be seen within the context of environmental involvement.

With specific regard to identity, Erikson attempted to integrate the theories of Freud on personality with James' discussion of 'character' formation to create a psychosocial theory of the individual's 'subjective sense of an invigorating sameness and continuity which is at issue in the various critical steps' or potential crises of his developmental model. Erikson's psychosocial propositions expand the psychoanalytic discussion. Yet Erikson remains firmly rooted in the psychoanalytic tradition, reforming rather than abandoning it. Indeed, Erikson's extensive discussion of identity continually bears the stamp of Freud's emphasis on the id's psychological ascendancy. It is to Erikson's credit that he incorporated environmental and historical factors into his psychoanalytic analysis of identity. Yet he continues to reckon with the individual's sense of continuity and character from the standpoint of the psychoanalytic observer which presupposes the causal priority of a 'psychological underworld.'

Succinctly put, previous treatments of identity can be criticized for attempting to elevate one single aspect of experience (social, biological, and/or psychological) to causal priority. No single component of identity-in-the-world can be said to 'cause' the others. Such an assertion would clearly abandon the dialectical character of lived experience and would lend an analytical simplicity that would lose the essential ambiguity of identity-in-the-world.

Traditional approaches to aging which have given priority to some unidimensional aspect of the experience of growing up and growing old have also forfeited the lived 'reality' of aging as it 'belongs to' people in daily life. Many treatments of aging have failed for reasons similar to those applied to the study of identity. Due to their common understanding of the individual as object, theories of aging have usually ignored aging as it is experienced and have rather focused on aging as a dimension of some social, psychological, or psychosocial model of reality. For the most part aging, and old age in particular, have been viewed in terms of 'stages.' This is to say that aging has been reduced to 'typical' stages of some objectively-assigned 'life cycle' (a phrase which itself implies a stage approach). The nature and content of these typical stages varies between the approaches, but the stage form, the objectification of aging, and the failure to account for aging as experienced remains in each perspective.

Among sociologists, for example, aging has often been treated as a phenomenon of macro analysis. This macro analysis of aging has in turn been largely informed by structural functionalism. As Davis and Moore have observed, the key problem upon which structural functional analysis has focused is how can a society 'distribute its members in social positions and induce them to perform the duties of these positions' (1945: 242)? It is in terms of this key societal problem that Linton (1942) introduced his seven age-sex statuses which are universally required for the purposes of classification and organization. Similarly, Parsons (1942) argued the import of the dual characteristics of age and sex for the structure of society. Eisenstadt (1956) provided one of the first thorough descriptions of 'age grading' and its central role in the 'continuity and stability' of the social system. Eisenstadt argued that age grading was essential to the division of labor, establishment of lines of seniority, definition of lines of authority in the family, economic, political, and occupational spheres. Cain (1964) also embraced and applauded Eisenstadt's thesis and cited its central import to overcoming 'biologistic' theories of aging. Typical of the approach, the effort to overcome 'biologistic' tendencies was so successful that aging became a totally disembodied phenomenon.

One of the more recent, while also the more comprehensive and articulate, statements of this same theme has been that of Riley, Johnson, and Foner (1972) on age stratification. As Riley *et al.* note, age stratification is based not on motivation but on the inevitable biological fact of aging. Still, rewards and prestige are allocated on the basis of age such that it remains an essential part of the social system. In accord with Eisenstadt, Riley *et al.* insist that aging differs from all other bases of stratification in its inevitable and irreversible nature (1972: 10). Nevertheless, as with other bases of stratification, aging is an important part of the structure of the social system and as such is essential to its continuity and stability.

It is indeed notable that Riley *et al.* recognize that the nature of aging is affected by many factors – psychological, social, as well as biological (1972: 10–11). They further recognize that aging 'belongs' to the individual (1972: 14). However, they fail to pursue this inherent complexity of aging, and consistently opt for an analysis of aging which examines it as the 'collective property of strata and cohorts' (1972: 14). In these terms their chief concerns lie with differences and lack of differences among age strata, size of strata (as processually affected by natality, mortality, and survival rates), life course differences in age cohorts, etc. Consequently, they never penetrate aging as it 'belongs' to the individual or is experienced, and they objectify that same experience by focusing on systemic needs.

Another pioneering attempt to theorize about aging, rooted in the structural functionalist tradition, is the now classic statement on 'disengagement theory' authored by Cumming and Henry (1961; see also Cumming *et al.* 1960). They are in basic agreement with Eisenstadt's assertion that aging constitutes 'one of the strongest, most essential links between the personality system of the individuals and the social system in which they participate' (1956: 32). Cumming and Henry's emphasis is on the equilibrium that must be maintained in society through internalized norms. As Cumming succinctly summarized their approach, 'normal aging is a mutual withdrawal or "disengagement" between the aging person and others in the social system to which he belongs – a withdrawal initiated by the individual himself or by others in the system' (1976: 20). To preserve continuity, the social system must force the elderly to disengage from economic, social, and familial roles. But this disengagement must take place in such a manner that the elderly actors, to maintain their own personality-system equilibrium, seek this same disengagement. Thus disengagement of individual and society is argued to be mutually satisfying.

Talcott Parsons embraced disengagement theory in his discussion of old age as the 'consummatory stage' of the life cycle (1963). He argued that it is a stage of 'harvest,' a time for the individual when 'the fruits of his previous instrumental commitments are primarily gathered in' (1963: 53). In short, passage to old age is a process by which the individual and society distance themselves from each other as a way to maintain the social system while rewarding the individual for a life well lived.

While disengagement theory attempts to provide a closer contact with the individual's encounter with the aging process than does the age stratification model, its emphasis remains on systemic needs. As with the age stratification theorists, disengagement theorists are primarily concerned with the maintenance of stability and continuity within the social system. Stability and continuity are maintained in the face of aging by the withdrawal of elderly actors from active social involvement. The systemic needs of the personality are also met for the elderly actor as her/his satisfaction is achieved through the 'sublimated enjoyment' of the surrogate activities of her/his children, financial security flowing from her/his own instrumental dedication to her/his work now finished, etc. As in the study of identity, the structural functionalist approach to aging, manifest in disengagement theory, remains preoccupied with the social while further over-mechanizing the experience of aging by defining it (as well as the social) in terms of system needs. Consciousness (or active self) and embodied experience are totally lost in the approach.

Various 'activity theories' have sprung from the symbolic interactionist tradition in part as a refutation of disengagement theory and in part as a logical extension of its guiding principles (see Rose 1968). While still maintaining the priority of the social, activity theorists have avoided the problematic assumption of societal equilibrium while emphasizing the need of people to engage actively in interaction with others in their social environment. Lemon *et al*. (1972) have suggested that the essential insight of the theory is a positive relationship between activity and life satisfaction such that the lower the level of activity, the lower the life satisfaction. Furthermore, life satisfaction is, in turn, positively related to self concept.

Since Havighurst and Albrecht's (1953) first explicit statement of this relationship between social participation and activity and life satisfaction, numerous other writers have utilized this framework to approach aging in both theoretical terms (Burgess 1950; Havighurst 1961; Cavan 1962; Rosow 1967; Howard Becker 1968 for examples) and in empirical studies (see Lebo 1953; Kutner *et al*. 1956; Reichard *et al*. 1962; Tobin and Neugarten 1961; Tallmer and Kutner 1970 for examples).

In contrast with the structural functionalist concentration on system needs and equilibrium, symbolic interactionists have emphasized the negotiated nature of age roles and statuses. This is to say that the individual is ascribed more room to maneuver than in the structural functionalist model. By avoiding a discussion of system needs, symbolic interactionists are able to stress individual needs for engagement rather than disengagement. Aging remains, however, a matter of social roles played – a 'career' of statuses. Age identity is even a matter of role definition (Rose 1968) tied largely to adult socialization processes (Rosow 1974). Old age poses a threat of the 'roleless role' (Burgess 1950), and even death has been portrayed as a status passage to the great 'roleless role' (Strauss 1969). In other words, both structural functionalist and symbolic interactionist approaches to aging have, in their overzealous and all-consuming affirmation of the social dimension of that phenomenon, ignored the subjective nature of aging as experienced by people in-the-world and they have further avoided the dynamics of physiological change implicit to the aging process (just as in the study of identity, both these approaches seem to have a dread fear of the specter of sociobiology). In this way they forsake the complexity of aging itself.

Another social psychological model of aging which is moored in the symbolic interactionist tradition, while more specifically concerned with labeling processes, discusses the 'social breakdown syndrome' (Kuypers and Bengston 1973; Bengston 1973). Kuypers and Bengston argue their central insight to be that 'an individual's sense of self, his ability to mediate between self and society and his orientation toward personal mastery are functions of the kinds of social labeling experienced in life' (1973: 181). They discuss old age as a stage characterized by declines in normative guidance, shrinkages of roles, and losses in appropriate reference groups. Such factors, they insist, make the individual vulnerable to the incompetent or deficient label which the wider society systematically applies. Ultimately, this notion of incompetence is internalized by the older person her/himself as the object of social labeling processes.

Again, with the social breakdown model, the person experiencing the

Appendix 2

aging process is less of a concern than is creating a model of that process. The end product is therefore often the portrayal of the individual as battered about by the labeling forces of society, an object of social forces which fail to account for issues pertinent to the individual's active embrace of experience.

Each of these theories of aging offers some insight into the experience of late life. Yet each, in one way or another, ignores the multifaceted nature of old age for the sake of theoretical or conceptual convenience. In an age of disciplinary specialization this may be expected but it can only be excused at the expense of an adequate (and accurate) understanding of what it means to grow old.

Sociologists haven't, of course, been the only ones to forfeit the complexity of aging in order to pursue the agenda of their theoretical models. The psychoanalytic approach to aging, for one, has taken several different forms but each tends to be subject to similar criticism. They have all shared in common, however, the need to go beyond Freud's discussion of the child's psychosexual development to account for the individual's move into postadolescent adulthood. Postchildhood development has long challenged the psychoanalytic approach precisely in the light of the psychosexual priority it has opted for in interpreting individual development. In childhood the libidinal energy of the id is seen as the driving force in development. With the exception of the 'degenerative' menopausal event for women, there is no further significant psychosexual crisis. In short, the libidinal energy of early psychic development is not extended into postchildhood development and as such the latter is wanting for explanation.

Freud himself chose to remain firm on the instinctual determinism at the root of both childhood and postchildhood development. Since development seems to peak in early adulthood, followed by a steady degeneration of the body through aging, he argued that there must be a second kind of instinctual drive, i.e. the 'death instinct.' It is the death instinct which, in Freud's words, 'seems more primitive, more elementary, more instinctual' than even the pleasure principle (1961: 17). For Freud, then, human aging is characterized by two opposing instinctual drives, one toward life and the other toward death. His thesis (only briefly touched upon in his own work) is that sexual life-forces have priority during early development but that the balance is tipped toward death instinct in later life.

Subsequent writers in the psychoanalytic tradition have attempted to articulate additional forces which might supplement Freud's original psychosexual theses to account better for development through the life cycle. One of the most notable in this regard has been Charlotte Buhler. Buhler embraces Freudian psychoanalytic principles, yet criticized Freud for not adequately dealing with human creativity (1959: 567; see also 1968: 18). She insists that there are four basic 'life tendencies' which represent a sort of ground plan for human development. These are:

1 need satisfaction;

145

2 adaptive self limitation;
3 creative expansion; and
4 upholding of internal order.

This belief in the four basic life tendencies has led Buhler and others to focus on what they believe to be the inverted U-shaped biological curve of life and psychological traits (Buhler 1968: 60; Frenkel-Brunswik 1968: 79). The four basic life tendencies tend to correspond roughly with biological changes in the organism. Young children are primarily concerned with need satisfaction. The older child begins the process of adaptive self-limitation. Carrying on then beyond the traditional psycho-analytic model, Buhler discusses adolescence and young adulthood as beginning the period of creative expansion. This marks a multidimensional period of life including such dramatic events as leaving home, choosing a vocation, marriage, and reproductivity. This period of creative expansion lasts until approximately age 40, when the maintenance of the internal order becomes a top priority. Buhler contends that from age 40 to the 60s 'the tendency to establish internal order becomes predominant' (1961: 366). It is a period marked by considerable self-assessment. Furthermore, Buhler insists that this struggle to establish internal order seems to be both a conscious and unconscious tendency (Buhler 1961: 368).

Buhler's model of biopsychological development in the process of aging has been further refined to include additional age categories (Buhler 1968: 14; Frenkel-Brunswik 1968) and further psychological specificity. The Freudian earmark remains apparent, however, and as such the individual seems to be at the mercy of biological growth/decline and the basic life tendencies of psychological development. Buhler's model shows relatively little concern for the social, and the narrow scope of human creativity outside a biopsychological determinism is apparent.

A second Freudian approach to aging is offered by Erik Erikson. He expands the original psychoanalytic model (as noted earlier in the discussion of identity) by attempting to psychosocialize Freud. Erikson accepts Freud's argument that the infant is 'all id' and that the driving force of early development is the sexual energy of the libido. Further he accepts Freud's contention that the child's early development is character-ized by a series of both internal and external conflicts. He attempts to expand Freud's thesis by insisting 'for man, to remain psychologically alive, must resolve these conflicts unceasingly' (1980: 52). Thus Erikson's key point of departure is to lend specificity to these conflicts continuing throughout the life cycle. Erikson suggests that there is an 'epigenetic principle' of eight stages of the life cycle, coinciding with eight psychosocial crises (see Erikson 1968, 1980). Infancy is characterized by the psychosocial crisis of trust versus mistrust, early childhood by autonomy versus shame and doubt, play age by initiative versus guilt, school age by industry versus inferiority, adolescence by identity versus diffusion, young adulthood by intimacy versus isolation, adulthood by generativity versus self absorption, mature age by integrity versus despair. Erikson explicitly hopes to dovetail psychosexual and psychosocial epigenesis (1980: 131) and his first six psychosocial crises closely coincide

Appendix 2

with Freudian psychosexual stages (see his worksheet in the appendix, Erikson 1980). It would be inappropriate to develop the entirety of Erikson's analysis here, but it should be noted that the period of adolescence represents a pivotal point within the framework. This is due to the fact that at this stage social developmental tasks of adult roles outweigh the biosexual developmental tasks of early maturation (1980: 94). Thus in the stage characterized by the psychological crisis of identity versus role diffusion, Erikson posits that biological priority begins to meld with a sort of social priority in adulthood. By so asserting, Erikson is able to see the possibility of personal growth into old age but does so only via this significant modification of the original Freudian thesis. He does so perhaps out of the need, shared by other neo-Freudians, to accomplish what Marcuse has called a 'revisionist combination of psychoanalysis with idealist ethics' (1955: 237). Thus, despite the usefulness of his concepts (integrity and despair) and the salience of some of his observations, Erikson's own theoretical agenda becomes more important than does the experience of aging by people in-the-world.

The preceding glimpse at previous theories of aging is intended only to allow us to arrive at the following point: when applied to theories of the life course, the approaches of symbolic interactionism, structural functionalism, and psychoanalysis all tend to objectify human experience. Not only do they make the individual the mere object of some unidimensional aspect of human experience but they also focus on their respective model of that experience. Indeed, the tendency to focus upon the latter ultimately leads to the error of the former. These theories of aging have thus emphasized aging as a series of stages, defining the process in terms of categories meaningful to the social scientific observer rather than in terms of aging as it is experienced by individual actors themselves. For symbolic interactionists aging is the product of labeling processes and role definitions. For structural functionalists aging is 'mobility from one age stratum to the next' ending in a disengagement process. For the psychoanalytic theorist aging is the multistaged balancing act of the ego in its confrontation with the conflicting instinctual drives of the libido and the death instinct or a melding of psychosexual and psychosocial crises. This isn't to say that these writers have nothing to say about human aging; on the contrary, they often capture critical insights into the experience. Yet to fail to appreciate the importance of the changing body, changing social networks, and people's psychological responses to these changes (that is, in relationship to one another), is to forfeit the true complexity of the aging experience. Aging, like identity, is always the intentional unity of individual consciousness (with all its projects, relevances, and purposes) acting upon an ever-changing organism and continually renegotiated social world. Inasmuch as aging constantly underlies the self appraisals of people engaged with the world, it is all the more appropriate to speak of age identity-in-the-world.

The flaws of previous treatments of human aging become clear in the empirical study of new vision loss which can accompany older age. The literature on blindness and people's experience of it can be subjected to

147

Appendix 2

similar criticism. While there have been relatively few explicit treatments
of identity and vision loss, there has been substantial relevant literature.
Not surprisingly, the treatments of vision loss in this regard have
paralleled the treatments of identity and aging reviewed earlier. In a
similar fashion, traditional approaches to vision loss and, more specifically,
blindness have relied on social scientific models of the blind or visually-
impaired person seen as the object of various psychobiological and social
forces. Thus in a like manner, treatments of blindness and visual impairment
have typically treated the theoretical constructs of the social scientist as the
reality of the phenonomen while forfeiting a grasp of the first-order
constructs of those people who actually live through vision loss. Again, as
with theories of aging, a cursory glimpse at these theories of blindness and
vision loss seems in order.

Treatments of blindness and vision impairment rooted in the psychoanalytic tradition have been well received by students of blindness over the
past several decades (for a full bibliographic review of this literature see
Bauman 1976) and are still enthusiastically embraced (see for example
Kirtley 1975). They have typically focused upon such factors as the sexual
symbolism of the eye, the resulting castration anxiety induced by the threat
of vision loss or upon the impact of blindness on normal psychosexual
development. The underlying assumption of these approaches has been that
such psychosexual factors, in large, explain the relationship of vision loss to
behavior (of both visually-impaired persons and sighted people's reactions).

Blank (1957) concisely summarized the symbolism of the eye which makes
blindness compelling to psychoanalytic interest. He insisted that the symbolic
import of the eye is rooted in its unconscious significance as a sexual organ
(including the equating of the eye with the mouth and with the genitals) or,
more specifically, as a hostile, destructive organ (including equating the eye
with 'piercing phallus' and 'devouring mouth'). This same symbolic
interchangeability of the eye and the phallus, in particular, has been recently
affirmed by Kirtley (1975: 31), citing such popular expressions as 'He
ravished her with his eyes,' 'He looked right through her,' 'She melted under
his gaze.' Kirtley further points to certain standard meanings of the word eye
that entail a connection between vision and projectile weaponry, such as 'to
eye' and 'to aim at' and 'eyeshot.' Both Blank and Kirtley simply reiterated
the earlier works of Schauer (1951), Braverman (1951), and Chevigny and
Braverman (1950) in this regard. These latter writers were specifically
concerned with describing the relationship of the eye's symbolism to the fear
sighted people have of themselves going blind and of interacting with others
who are already blind.

This central psychoanalytic presupposition of the eye's phallic significance
has led writers in this tradition to focus on 'castration anxieties' that
accompany the loss of sight. Braverman, for example, concludes that 'we
find that most of the attitudes toward the blind and the misconceived beliefs
on which those attitudes are based, can be understood in terms of the
castration anxiety' that accompanies the loss of sight (1951: 145). In other
words, attitudes toward blindness and the blind flow from the castration fears
which are mobilized by the loss of sight (again equated with phallic

148

significance). Chevigny and Braverman (1950) amass considerable literary, historical, and clinical 'evidence' regarding this relationship between attitudes and castration fears: from literature, Milton's Samson Agonistes likens himself to a 'castrated ram'; from history, blindness was used for the purposes of 'symbolic' castration in punishment for sexual offenses; in clinical circles, schizophrenic males are reported to mutilate their eyes in self-reprisal for imagined sexual transgressions. These and many other cases from all three sources convince Chevigny and Braverman that most attitudes toward blindness (sometimes shared by blind persons themselves, see Kirtley's clinical examples, 1975: 31ff.) are rooted in the belief that the loss of sight correlates with sexual ineffectiveness. Not only does this castration anxiety produce fear of losing one's own sight but it also prompts reactions of revulsion, guilt, anxiety, and pity when the sighted are forced to confront blindness in others (Braverman 1951: 157). This is argued to be particularly troubling for parents of blind children (Blank 1957: 5).

The psychoanalytic approach to blindness has also been concerned with its effect upon the psychosexual development of ego functioning. Carl Davis, for example, insists that problems of 'differentiation' often result for children who are blind (1964). As he describes the process in the 'normal' child, it is through the use of vision that individuals are initially enabled to perceive that their mother and other individuals are not part of them, that there are many other objects (crib extending outwards) in their environment which are not part of them either. Vision, then, allows a child to differentiate her/himself from her/his environment. Davis further asserts that vision allows a child to begin to forge a mental image of her/his structure. These processes are disturbed (but hopefully only delayed) in the blind child (a concern also voiced by Blank 1957: 7). Thomas Cutsforth (1933) insisted that such limitations on the personality development of blind children led to their being generally neurotic and often sexually maladjusted. Ultimately, Cutsforth argued that blind people develop such traits as passivity, egocentricity, submissiveness, and sexual maladjustment. (Note that neither Bauman 1954 nor Cowen *et al.* 1961 were able to confirm Cutsforth's notion of the 'neurotic blind personality.')

By similar reasoning, new vision loss for individuals with fully-developed ego functioning has been argued to be potentially traumatic as well (Blank 1957: 11). Blank suggests that new vision loss leads to a sort of 'depersonalization' of the individual in which the old personality is held in abeyance (acting as a sort of 'protective emotional anesthesia'). He argues that the concept of 'rebirth' of the blind person is essential (1957: 13) because new vision loss forces a new period of infancy and childhood in which many psychosexual aspects of development are recreated and the potential for personality disorders revived.

In contrast with psychoanalytic treatments of blindness and vision loss, Lukoff and Whiteman observe that a second major trend has emerged which focuses upon the social milieu in which visually-impaired persons find themselves enmeshed (1970: 15). Here social milieu is given priority over and against psychosexual considerations. Lukoff and Whiteman's own treatment of the social forces influencing the adaptation of blind persons to

Appendix 2

their social roles and socialization processes in their *Social Sources of Adjustment to Blindness* (1970) is one of the most comprehensive attempts to catalog this same milieu. Lukoff and Whiteman focused upon Linton's distinction between status and role, attempting to describe, then, the obligations attributed to the position of blind persons within society and the ways in which they carry out their status (1970: 42ff.). Correspondingly, they concentrated on the perceived expectations of family, sighted friends, blind friends, and employers, as well as the standards of performance blind persons hold for themselves in view of these perceived expectations (1970: 50). Lukoff and Whiteman thus argue that their study of 498 people who were blind demonstrated that internalized self-standards are, in large part, determined by the perceived expectations of their primary relationships with those who share similar value perspectives. Various socioeconomic variables were further argued to determine these same commonly-shared value perspectives; social class, race, ethnicity, education were all considered as important variables in setting normative standards for blind persons. Lukoff and Whiteman argue that it is impossible to speak of the personality of the individual who is blind but insist, rather, that the blind person, like any other, faces a heterogeneous set of orientations.

The Lukoff and Whiteman study endorsed and expanded upon the earlier work of such writers as Alan Gowman (1957), whose study of war-blinded veterans showed that stereotypical misconceptions of blindness block opportunities for them to engage in reciprocal relations with sighted people. These same reduced opportunities were argued by Gowman to distort the blind person's sense of self and situation in life such that uniformities in blind 'personalities' actually emerge from common reactions to these limitations placed upon them. Similarly, Josephson (1968) has suggested that blind people can only be adequately understood in terms of their opportunities in leisure, education, employment, and living arrangements. He further argued that 'the growth of special institutions for the blind has in some respects tended to segregate those who are most dependent on the agencies for their education, employment and recreation' (1968: 82). This isolation gives them a sort of minority group status which dictates both their opportunities and their ensuing behavior.

Common to the treatments of vision loss by Gowman, Josephson, Lukoff, and Whiteman is the assumption that blindness must be understood in terms of people's positions within society, which then induces them to perform the corresponding duties of that location. Here they are all consistent with the structural functionalist presuppositions voiced by Parsons, Davis, and Moore, and others reviewed in the earlier discussions of identity and aging.

Directly pertinent to the concern with identity, other writers on blindness and vision impairment have focused on the insights of symbolic interactionism and attempt to stress that one's conception of situation and character is the product of the stigmatized labels applied by those around him/her. Erving Goffman, for example, relied heavily upon the blind to demonstrate his thesis in *Stigma* (1963). Citing blindness as an instance of stigma resulting from 'abominations of the body,' Goffman argues that it has the effect (as do other forms of stigma) that 'an individual who might have been received easily in ordinary social intercourse possesses a trait that can obtrude itself upon attention and turn those of us whom he meets away from him' (1963: 5). By definition blind persons are treated as being not quite human, contaminated, discredited, indeed threatening to so-called 'normals,' and are finally victimized by these conceptions of their situation. The blind person, argues Goffman, forges her/his very 'ego identity' (subjective sense of situation, continuity, and character – the lived identity of the present study) from these preconceptions of those around her/him. Goffman insists 'the individual constructs his image of himself out of the same materials from which others first construct a social and personal identification of him' (1963: 106). While Goffman allows stigmatized individuals 'important liberties' in terms of what they fashion from the conceptions of those in their immediate social environment, the blind person's sense of self is primarily defined by the labels supplied by 'normals' and the mutual affirmation of her/his abnormality by fellow members within the stigmatized group (her/his 'real group' – Goffman 1963: 113).

Similarly, Robert Scott in his *Making of Blind Men* argues that 'the substance of a man's self image consists of his perceptions of the evaluations that others make of him and particularly those of others whose opinions he values most highly' (1969: 15). Scott continues by asserting that a blind person's sense of self, like other people, is 'made' through the process of socialization beginning early in and continuing throughout her/his life. Blindness is thus a learned social role. Preconceptions about blindness (blind people are helpless, dependent, incapacitated, etc.) become a reality for a blind person. Scott argues that they are acquired in the blind person's intercourse with sighted people, other individuals who are blind, and with the service agencies aimed at their 'rehabilitation.' The commonalities shared by blind persons are the product of the persistent application of these stigmatizing preconceptions through socialization processes which tend to reward behavior consistent with them and discourage deviations from them. The blind person thus becomes a member of a group of people 'who initially share in common only the fact that they have problems of vision and eventually come to feel and behave in patterned, predictable ways' (Scott 1969: 120–1).

Many of the labeling presuppositions of Goffman's and Scott's interactionist treatments of blindness and vision loss have been suspiciously received by practitioners and other writers in the field alike (in the case of the latter see, for example, Lukoff's cricitism of the approach 1972: 22). Nevertheless, it is notably to their credit that they begin to return the examination of blindness from preoccupations with either unconscious psychosexual drives or issues of mere social placement back to the level of the lived experience of blind actors themselves. Their contribution in this regard cannot be minimized. Their accounts are not allowed, however, to carry this examination of lived experience to full fruition as they both remain preoccupied with demonstrating the utility of the symbolic interactionist framework which unfortunately excludes other pertinent aspects of vision loss-in-the world.

When applied to the phenomenon of vision loss, the approaches of psychoanalysis, structural functionalism, and symbolic interactionism end up objectifying human experience, each in their unique way, just as they did when their models were used to explore identity and aging. The 'reality' of vision loss again becomes the 'reality' as it appears to the social scientist, tempered by his or her own theoretical and methodological agenda. For the psychoanalytic theorist vision loss is the mobilization of castration anxieties in both blind and sighted alike. For structural functionalists vision loss is a status within a social system with correspond-ing normative standards for behavior. For the symbolic interactionist vision loss is the stigma produced through labeling processes and role definitions. Just as in the treatments of identity and aging, these three traditional approaches to vision loss all tend to make the individual an object of various psychobiological and social forces, thus forfeiting the full complexity of vision loss as it is lived. Again, it is not so much that these authors have nothing to say – quite the contrary, many of them have a great deal to offer by way of insight into various aspects of the experience of blindness and vision loss. And yet, just as with traditional theories of aging (and even theories of identity more generally), they have avoided the necessary complexity (and one could add necessary ambiguity) of people's experience.

Bibliography

Adams, George and Pearlman, Jerome (1970) 'Emotional response and
  management of visually handicapped patients,' *Psychiatry in Medicine*
  1: 233–40.
Ainlay, Stephen and Crosby, Faye (1986) 'Stigma, justice and the
  dilemma of difference,' in Stephen Ainlay, Gaylene Becker, and
  Lerita Coleman (eds) *The Dilemma of Difference*, New York: Plenum.
Ainlay, Stephen and Redfoot, Donald (1982) 'Aging and identity-in-the-
  world: a phenomenological analysis,' *International Journal of Aging
  and Human Development* 15: 1–16.
Altshuler, K. (1970) 'Reaction to and management of sensory loss:
  blindness and deafness,' in Bernard Schoenberg, Arthur Carr, and
  David Peretz (eds) *Loss and Grief: Psychological Management in
  Medical Practice*, New York: Columbia University Press.
Angell, Robert (1945) 'A critical review of the development of personal
  document method in sociology, 1920–1940,' in Louis Gottschalk,
  Clyde Kluckhohn, and Robert Angell, *The Use of Personal Documents
  in History, Anthropology and Sociology*, New York: Social Science
  Research Council.
Argyle, Michael (1969) *Social Interaction*, New York: Atherton Press.
Argyle, Michael and Dean, Janet (1973) 'Eye contact, distance and
  affiliation,' in Michael Argyle (ed.) *Social Encounters*, Chicago:
  Aldine.
Atchley, Robert (1985) *Social Forces and Aging*, Belmont, CA:
  Wadsworth.
Back, Kurt and Gergen, Kenneth (1968) 'The self through the later span
  of life,' in Chad Gordon and Kenneth Gergen (eds) *The Self in Social
  Interaction*, New York: Wiley.
Baker, Larry Dale (1973) 'Blindness and social behavior: a need for
  research,' *New Outlook for the Blind* 67: 315–18.
Baldwin, Alfred (1961) 'The Parsonian theory of the personality,' in Max
  Black (ed.) *The Social Theories of Talcott Parsons*, Carbondale, IL:
  Southern Illinois University Press.
Barker, Roger with Wright, Beatrice and Gonick, Mollie (1953)
  *Adjustment to Physical Handicap and Illness: A Survey of the Social
  Psychology of Physique and Disability*, New York: Social Science
  Research Council.

Bauman, Mary (1954) *Adjustment to Blindness*, Pennsylvania: Pennsylvania State Council for the Blind.

Bauman, Mary (1976) *Blindness, Visual Impairment, Deaf-Blindness: Annotated Listing of the Literature 1953–75*, Philadelphia: Temple University Press.

Beauvoir, Simone de (1972) *The Coming of Age*, New York: G.P. Putnam's Sons.

Becker, Ernest (1973) *The Denial of Death*, New York: Free Press.

Becker, Gaylene (1980) *Growing Old in Silence*, Berkeley: University of California Press.

Becker, Howard (1963) *Outsiders*, Glencoe, IL: Free Press.

Becker, Howard (1966) 'Introduction' to Clifford Shaw, *The Jack Roller*, Chicago: University of Chicago Press, 1930.

Becker, Howard (1968) 'Personal change in adult life,' in Bernice Neugarten (ed.) *Middle Age and Aging*, Chicago: University of Chicago Press.

Benedek, T. (1952) 'Personality development,' in F. Alexander and H. Ross (eds) *Dynamic Psychiatry*, Chicago: University of Chicago Press.

Bengston, Vern (1973) *The Social Psychology of Aging*, Indianapolis: Bobbs-Merrill.

Berger, Peter (1966) 'On existential phenomonology and sociology,' *American Sociological Review* 31: 259–60.

Berger, Peter (1967) *The Sacred Canopy*, Garden City, NY: Anchor/Doubleday.

Berger, Peter (1970) 'Identity as a problem in the sociology of knowledge,' in James Curtis and John Petras (eds) *The Sociology of Knowledge*, New York: Praeger.

Berger, Peter with Berger, Brigette and Kellner, Hansfried (1973) *The Homeless Mind*, New York: Random House.

Berger, Peter and Kellner, Hansfried (1981) *Sociology Reinterpreted: An Essay on Method and Vocation*, Garden City, NY: Anchor/Doubleday.

Berger, Peter and Luckmann, Thomas (1966) *The Social Construction of Reality*, New York: Anchor/Doubleday.

Bernstein, Norman (1975) *Emotional Care of the Facially Burned and Disfigured*, Boston: Little, Brown & Co.

Birdwhistell, Ray (1970) *Kinesics and Context*, Philadelphia: University of Pennsylvania Press.

Birdwhistell, Ray (1973) 'Kinesics,' in Michael Argyle (ed.) *Social Encounters*, Chicago: Aldine.

Birren, James (1963) 'Psychosociological relations,' in J. Birren, R. Butler, S. Greenhouse, L. Sokoloff, and M. Yarrow (eds) *Human Aging: A Biological and Behavioral Study*, Washington, DC: US Government Printing Office.

Blank, H. Robert (1957) 'Psychoanalysis and blindness,' *Psychoanalytic Quarterly* 26: 1–24.

Bogdan, Robert and Taylor, Steven (1975) *Introduction to Qualitative Research Methods*, New York: Wiley.

Braverman, Sydell (1951) 'Psychological roots of attitudes toward blindness,' *New Outlook for the Blind* 45: 151–7.

Brooks, Karen and Dunn, Susan (1974) 'Dancers in Darkness,' *Journal of School Health* 44: 147–51.

Bruner, Jerome (1987) 'Life as narrative,' *Social Research* 54: 11–32.

Buhler, Charlotte (1959) 'Theoretical observations about life's basic tendencies,' *American Journal of Psychotherapy* 13: 561–81.

Buhler, Charlotte (1961) 'Meaningful living in the mature years,' in Robert Kleemeir (ed.) *Aging and Leisure*, New York: Oxford University Press.

Buhler, Charlotte (1968) 'The general structure of the human life cycle,' in Charlotte Buhler and Fred Massarik (eds) *The Course of Human Life*, New York: Springer.

Buhler, Charlotte and Goldenberg, Herbert (1968) 'Structural aspects of the individual's history,' in Charlotte Buhler and Fred Massarik (eds) *The Course of Human Life*, New York: Springer.

Burgess, Ernest (1950) 'Personal and social adjustment in old age,' in Milton Derber (ed.) *Aged and Society*, Champaign, IL: Industrial Relations Press.

Burgess, Ernest (1966) 'Discussion,' in Clifford Shaw, *The Jack Roller*, Chicago: University of Chicago Press.

Butler, Robert (1968) 'The life review: an interpretation of reminiscence in the aged,' in Bernice Neugarten (ed.) *Middle Age and Aging*, Chicago: University of Chicago Press.

Butler, Robert and Lewis, Myrna (1977) *Aging and Mental Health*, St Louis: C.V. Mosby.

Cain, Leonard (1964) 'Life course and social structure,' in R.L. Faris (ed.) *Handbook of Modern Sociology*, Chicago: Rand-McNally.

Cavan, Ruth (1962) 'Self and role in adjustment during old age,' in Arnold Rose (ed.) *Human Behavior and Social Processes*, Boston: Houghton Mifflin.

Chalkley, Thomas (1974) *Your Eyes*, Springfield, IL: Charles Thomas.

Charme, Stuart (1984) *Meaning and Myth in the Study of Lives*, Philadelphia: University of Pennsylvania Press.

Chevigny, Hector (1946) *My Eyes Have a Cold Nose*, New Haven: Yale University Press.

Chevigny, Hector and Braverman, Sydell (1950) *The Adjustment of the Blind*, New Haven: Yale University Press.

Choisy, Maryse (1963) *Sigmund Freud: A New Appraisal*, New York: Philosophical Library.

Cicourel, Aron (1964) *Method and Measurement in Sociology*, New York: Free Press.

Cicourel, Aron (1974) *Cognitive Sociology*, New York: Free Press.

Clark, Margaret and Anderson, Barbara (1967) *Culture and Aging*, Springfield, IL: Charles Thomas.

Clausen, John (1972) 'The life course of individuals,' in Matilda Riley, Marilyn Johnson, and Anne Foner (eds) *Aging and Society, Volume*

Three: A Sociology of Age Stratification, New York: Russell Sage Foundation.

Coni, Nicholas with Davidson, William and Webster, Stephen (1977) *Lecture Notes on Geriatrics*, Oxford: Blackwell.

Cowen, Emery with Verillo, Ronald, Underberg, Rita, and Benham, F. (1961) *Adjustment to Visual Disability in Adolescents*, New York: American Foundation for the Blind.

Cumming, Elaine (1976) 'Further thoughts on the theory of disengagement,' in Cary Kart and Barbara Manard (eds) *Aging in America*, Sherman Oaks, CA: Alfred Publishing.

Cumming, Elaine with Dean, Lois, Newell, David, and McCaffrey, Isabel (1960) 'Disengagement: a tentative theory of aging,' *Sociometry* 23: 23–35.

Cumming, Elaine and William, Henry (1961) *Growing Old*, New York: Basic Books.

Curle, Adam (1972) *Mystics and Militants*, London: Tavistock.

Cutler, Neal and Harootyan, Robert (1975) 'Demography of the aged,' in Diana Woodruff and James Birren (eds) *Aging*, New York: Van Nostrand.

Cutsforth, Thomas (1933) *The Blind in School and Society*, New York: American Foundation for the Blind.

Davidson, Helen and Lang, Gerhard (1960) 'Children's perceptions of their teachers' feelings toward them related to self perception, school achievement and behavior,' *Journal of Experimental Education* 29: 107–18.

Davis, Carl (1964) 'Development of the self concept,' *New Outlook for the Blind* 58: 49–51.

Davis, Fred (1963) *Passage Through Crisis*, Indianapolis: Bobbs-Merrill.

Davis, Fred (1964) 'Deviance disavowal: the management of strained interaction by the visibly handicapped,' in Howard Becker (ed.) *The Other Side*, New York: Free Press.

Davis, Kingsley and Moore, Wilbert (1945) 'Some principles of stratification,' *American Sociological Review*: 242–9.

Denzin, Norman (1970) *The Research Act*, Chicago: Aldine.

Douglas, Jack (1970) *Understanding Everyday Life*, Chicago: Aldine.

Dover, Francis (1959) 'Readjusting to the onset of blindness,' *Social Casework*, 40: 334–8.

Eden, John (1978) *The Eye Book*, Harmondsworth: Penguin.

Eisenstadt, S.N. (1956) *From Generation to Generation: Age Groups and Social Structure*, Glencoe, IL: Free Press.

Erikson, Erik (1950) *Childhood and Society*, New York: Norton.

Erikson, Erik (1968) *Identity: Youth and Crisis*, New York: Norton.

Erikson, Erik (1980) *Identity and the Life Cycle*, New York: The International Universities Press.

Erikson, Kai (1962) 'Notes on the sociology of deviance,' *Social Problems* 9: 311–12.

Faraday, Annabel and Plummer, Kenneth (1979) 'Doing life histories,' *Sociological Review* 27: 773–98.

Finch, Caleb and Hayflick, Leonard (1977) *The Handbook of the Biology of Aging*, New York: Van Nostrand, Reinhold.

Fischer, David H. (1978) *Growing Old in America*, New York: Oxford University Press.

Fisher, Seymour (1973) *Body Consciousness*, Englewood Cliffs, NJ: Prentice-Hall.

Fisher, Seymour and Cleveland, Sidney (1968) *Body Image and Personality*, New York: Dover.

Fitzgerald, Roy (1971) 'Visual phenomenology in recently blind adults,' *American Journal of Psychiatry* 127: 1,533–9.

Foulke, Emerson (1972) 'The personality of the blind: an invalid concept,' *New Outlook for the Blind* 66: 33–7, 42.

Freedman, Saul (1965) 'Reactions to blindness,' *New Outlook for the Blind* 59: 344–6.

Freeman, Joseph (1965) *Clinical Features of the Older Patient*, Springfield, IL: Charles Thomas.

Freeman, Mark (1984) 'History, narrative and life-span developmental knowledge,' *Human Development* 27: 1–19.

Frenkel-Brunswik, Else (1968) 'Adjustments and reorientation in the course of the life span,' in Bernice Neugarten (ed.) *Middle Age and Aging*, Chicago: University of Chicago Press.

Freud, Sigmund (1935) *A General Introduction to Psychoanalysis*, New York: Washington Square Press.

Freud, Sigmund (1952) *New Introductory Lectures on Psychoanalysis* from Great Books of the Western World, volume 54, Chicago: Encyclopedia Britannica.

Freud, Sigmund (1953) *Three Essays on the Theory of Sexuality*, London: Hogarth Press.

Freud, Sigmund (1960) *The Ego and the Id*, New York: Norton.

Freud, Sigmund (1961) *Beyond the Pleasure Principle*, New York: Norton.

Friedenwald, J.S. (1952) 'The eye,' in A. I. Lansing (ed.) *Cowdry's Problems of Aging*, Baltimore: Williams & Wilkins.

Garfinkel, Harold (1956) 'Conditions for successful degradation ceremonies,' *American Journal of Sociology* 61: 420–4.

Geertz, Clifford (1973) *The Interpretation of Culture*, New York: Harper & Row.

Goffman, Erving (1957) 'Alienation from interaction,' *Human Relations* 10: 47–60.

Goffman, Erving (1959) *The Presentation of Self in Everyday Life*, New York: Anchor/Doubleday.

Goffman, Erving (1961) *Asylums*, New York: Doubleday.

Goffman, Erving (1963) *Stigma*, Englewood Cliffs, NJ: Prentice-Hall.

Gowman, Alan (1957) *The War Blind in American Social Structure*, New York: American Foundation for the Blind.

Gurwitsch, Aron (1974) *Phenomenology and the Theory of Science*, Evanston, IL: Northwestern University Press.

Bibliography

Halasa, Adnan (1972) *The Basic Aspects of the Glaucomas*, Springfield, IL: Charles Thomas.

Hall, Edward (1959) *The Silent Language*, New York: Doubleday.

Hall, Edward (1966) *The Hidden Dimension*, New York: Doubleday.

Havighurst, Robert (1961) 'Successful aging,' *Gerontologist* 1: 8–13.

Havighurst, Robert and Albrecht, R. (1953) *Older People*, New York: Longmans, Green.

Hazell, Kenneth (1960) *Social and Medical Problems of the Elderly*, London: Hutchinson Medical Publications.

Husserl, Edmund (1970) *Cartesian Meditations*, The Hague: Martinus Nijhoff.

Jernigan, Kenneth (1965) 'Blindness: handicap or characteristic,' *New Outlook for the Blind* 59: 244–9.

Jervis, Frederick (1964) 'The self in process of obtaining and maintaining self esteem,' *New Outlook for the Blind* 58: 51–4.

Josephson, Eric (1968) *The Social Life of Blind People*, New York: American Foundation for the Blind.

Kasper, Robert (1983) 'Eye problems of the aged,' in William Reichel (ed.) *Clinical Aspects of Aging*, 2nd edition, Baltimore: Williams & Wilkins.

Kaufman, Sharon (1986) *The Ageless Self: Sources of Meaning in Late Life*, New York: New American Library.

Kendon, Adam (1973) 'Some functions of gaze-direction in social interaction,' in Michael Argyle, *Social Encounters*, Chicago: Aldine.

Kipnis, Dorothy (1961) 'Changes in self concept in relation to perception of others,' *Journal of Personality* 29: 449–65.

Kirchner, Corinne and Lowman, Cherry (1978) 'Sources of variation in the estimated prevalence of visual loss,' *Journal of Visual Impairment and Blindness* 72: 329–33.

Kirchner, Corinne and Peterson, Richard (1979) 'Statistical briefs: latest data on visual disability from NCHS,' *Journal of Visual Impairment and Blindness* 73: 151–3.

Kirtley, Donald (1975) *The Psychology of Blindness*, Chicago: Nelson Hall.

Kleck, Robert with Hiroshi, Ono and Hastorf, Albert (1966) 'The effects of physical deviance upon face-to-face interaction,' *Human Relations* 19: 425–36.

Koestler, Frances (1976) *The Unseen Minority*, New York: David McKay.

Kornzweig, Abraham (1979) 'The eye in old age,' in Isadore Rossman (ed.) *Clinical Geriatrics*, Philadelphia: Lippincott.

Kubler-Ross, Elisabeth (1975) *Death: The Final Stage of Growth*, Englewood Cliffs, NJ: Prentice-Hall.

Kuhn, Manford and McPartland, Thomas (1954) 'An empirical investigation of self-attitudes,' *American Sociological Review* 19: 68–76.

Kutner, Bernary with Fanshell, D., Togo, A., and Langer, S. (1956) *Five Hundred Over Sixty*, New York: Russell Sage Foundation.

Kuypers, J.A. and Bengston, Vern (1973) 'Competence and social breakdown: a social-psychological view of aging,' *Human Development* 16: 181–201.

Laing, R.D. (1960) *The Divided Self*, Harmondsworth: Penguin.

Lebo, D. (1953) 'Some factors said to make for happiness in old age,' *Journal of Clinical Psychology* 9: 384–90.

Lemon, Bruce with Bengston, Vern and Peterson, James (1972) 'An exploration of the activity theory of aging: activity types and life satisfaction among in-movers to a retirement community,' in Cary Kart and Barbara Manard (eds) *Aging in America*, Sherman Oaks, CA: Alfred Publishing.

Linton, Ralph (1942) 'Age and sex characteristics,' *American Sociological Review* 7: 589–603.

Lofland, John (1969) *Deviance and Identity*, Englewood Cliffs, NJ: Prentice-Hall.

Lukoff, Irving (1972) 'Psychosocial research and severe vision impairment,' in Milton Graham (ed.) *Science and Blindness*, New York: American Foundation for the Blind.

Lukoff, Irving and Whiteman, Martin (1970) *The Social Sources of Adjustment to Blindness*, New York: American Foundation for the Blind Research Series no. 121.

Manney, James (1975) *Aging in American Society*, Ann Arbor, MI: University of Michigan Press.

Marcuse, Herbert (1955) *Eros and Civilization*, New York: Random House.

Matza, David (1969) *Becoming Deviant*, Englewood Cliffs, NJ: Prentice-Hall.

Mead, George Herbert (1934) *Mind, Self and Society*, Chicago: University of Chicago Press.

Mead, George Herbert (1938) *The Philosophy of the Act*, Chicago: University of Chicago Press.

Mead, George Herbert (1964) 'Social consciousness and consciousness of meaning,' in Andrew Reck (ed.) *Selected Writings*, Indianapolis: Bobbs-Merrill.

Mehrabian, Albert (1973) 'Inference of attitudes from posture, orientation and distance of the communicator,' in Michael Argyle (ed.) *Social Encounters*, Chicago: Aldine.

Merleau-Ponty, Maurice (1962) *The Phenomenology of Perception*, New York: Routledge & Kegan Paul.

Merleau-Ponty, Maurice (1963) *The Structure of Behavior*, Boston, MA: Beacon Press.

Merleau-Ponty, Maurice (1964a) *Signs*, Evanston, IL: Northwestern University Press.

Merleau-Ponty, Maurice (1964b) 'The child's relations with others,' in his *The Primacy of Perception*, James Edie (ed.), Evanston, IL: Northwestern University Press.

Merleau-Ponty, Maurice (1970) *Themes from the Lectures*, Evanston, IL: Northwestern University Press.

Bibliography

Milton, John (1969) *Poetical Works*, Douglas Bush (ed.), Oxford: Oxford University Press.
Monbeck, Michael (1973) *The Meaning of Blindness*, Bloomington, IN: Indiana University Press.
Mykelbust, Helmer (1964) *The Psychology of Deafness: Sensory Deprivation, Learning and Adjustment*, New York: Grune & Stratton.
Natanson, Maurice (1970) *The Journeying Self*, Reading, MA: Addison Wesley.
Neu, Carlos (1975) 'Coping with newly diagnosed blindness,' *American Journal of Nursing* 75: 2,161–3.
O'Neill, John (1973) 'Embodiment and child development: a phenomenological approach,' in Hans Dreitzel (ed.) *Childhood and Socialization*, New York: Macmillan.
Oyer, Herbert and Oyer, Jane (1976) *Aging and Communication*, Baltimore: University Park Press.
Parsons, John (1970) *Diseases of the Eye*, London: Churchill Livingstone.
Parsons, Talcott (1942) 'Age and sex in the social structure of the United States,' *American Sociological Review* 7: 604–16.
Parsons, Talcott (1951) *The Social System*, Glencoe, IL: Free Press.
Parsons, Talcott (1963) 'Old age as a consummatory phase,' *Gerontologist* 3: 35–43.
Parsons, Talcott (1964) *Social Structure and Personality*, New York: Free Press.
Parsons, Talcott (1968) 'The position of identity in the general theory of action,' in Chad Gordon and Kenneth Gergen (eds) *The Self in Social Interaction*, New York: Wiley.
Peterson, Richard, Lowman, Cherry, and Kirchner, Corinne (1978) 'Visual handicap: statistical data on a social process,' *Journal of Visual Impairment and Blindness* 72: 419–21.
Potok, Andrew (1980) *Ordinary Daylight*, New York: Holt, Rinehart & Winston.
Psathas, George (1968) 'Ethnomethods and phenomenology,' *Social Research* 35: 500–20.
Psathas, George (1973) *Phenomenological Sociology: Issues and Applications*, New York: Wiley.
Reichard, Suzanne with Livson, F. and Peterson, P. (1962) *Aging and Personality*, New York: Wiley.
Richardson, Stephen with Dohrenwend, Barbara and Klein, David (1965) *Interviewing: Its Forms and Functions*, New York: Basic Books.
Riffenburgh, Ralph (1967) 'The psychology of blindness,' *Geriatrics* 22: 127–33.
Riley, Matilda and Foner, Anne, *et al.* (1968) *Aging and Society, Volume I*, New York: Russell Sage Foundation.
Riley, Matilda with Johnson, Marilyn and Foner, Anne (1972) *Aging and Society, Volume III: A Sociology of Age Stratification*, New York: Russell Sage Foundation.
Rose, Arnold (1961) 'Mental health of normal older persons,' *Geriatrics* 16: 459–64.

Rose, Arnold (1968) 'A current theoretical issue in social gerontology,' in Bernice Neugarten (ed.) *Middle Age and Aging*, Chicago: University of Chicago Press.

Rosow, Irving (1967) *Social Integration of the Aged*, New York: Free Press.

Rosow, Irving (1973) 'The social context of the aging self,' *The Gerontologist* 13: 82–7.

Rosow, Irving (1974) *Socialization to Old Age*, Berkeley: University of California Press.

Sartre, Jean-Paul (1953) *Being and Nothingness*, New York: Washington Square Press.

Saul, Shura (1983) *Aging: An Album of People Growing Old*, New York: Wiley.

Schauer, Gerhard (1951) 'Motivation of attitudes toward blindness,' *New Outlook for the Blind* 45: 39–42.

Scheie, Harold and Albert, Daniel (1969) *Adler's Textbook of Ophthalmology*, Philadelphia: Saunders.

Scheler, Max (1970) 'Lived body, environment and ego,' in Stuart Spicker (ed.) *The Philosophy of the Body*, New York: Quadrangle Books.

Schutz, Alfred (1971) *Collected Papers I: The Problem of Social Reality*, The Hague: Martinus Nijhoff.

Schutz, Alfred and Luckmann, Thomas (1973) *The Structures of the Life-World*, Evanston, IL: Northwestern University Press.

Schwartz, Barry (1975) *Queuing and Waiting*, Chicago: University of Chicago Press.

Schwartz, Barry (1978) 'The social ecology of time barriers,' *Social Forces* 56: 1,203–20.

Scott, Robert (1969) *The Making of Blind Men*, New York: Russell Sage Foundation.

Shontz, Franklin (1975) *The Psychological Aspects of Physical Illness and Disability*, New York: Macmillan.

Siller, Jerome with Ferguson, Linda, Vann, Donald, and Holland, Bert (1967) *Structure of Attitudes Toward the Physically Disabled*, New York: New York University Press.

Simmel, Georg (1970) 'On visual interaction,' in Gregory Stone and Harvey Farberman (eds), *Social Psychology Through Symbolic Interaction*, Waltham, MA: Xerox College Publishing.

Stafford, Mark and Scott, Richard (1986) 'Stigma, deviance and social control,' in Stephen Ainlay, Gaylene Becker, and Lerita Coleman (eds) *The Dilemma of Difference*, New York: Plenum.

Stone, Gregory (1962) 'Appearance and the self,' in Arnold Rose (ed.) *Human Behavior and Social Process*, Boston: Houghton Mifflin.

Strauss, Anselm (1969) *Mirrors and Masks*, Mill Valley, CA: The Sociology Press.

Tallmer, M. and Kutner, Bernard (1970) 'Disengagement and morale,' *Gerontologist* 10: 317–20.

Tobin, Sheldon and Neugarten, Bernice (1961) 'Life satisfaction and social interaction in the aging,' *Journal of Gerontology* 16: 344–6.

Bibliography

Toch, Hans (1955) 'Crisis situations and ideological evaluations,' *Public Opinion Quarterly* 19: 53–67.

Treas, Judith (1975) 'Aging and the family,' in Diana Woodruff and James Birren (eds) *Aging: Scientific Perspectives and Social Issues*, New York: Van Nostrand.

Truzzi, Marcello (1968) 'Lilliputians in Gulliver's Land: the social role of the dwarf,' in his *Sociology and Everyday Life*, Englewood Cliffs, NJ: Prentice-Hall.

Van Weelden, Jacob (1967) *On Being Blind*, Amsterdam: Netherlands Society for the Blind.

Veirs, Everett (1970) *So You Have Glaucoma?* New York: Grune & Stratton.

Weigert, Andrew (1975) 'Substantival self: a primitive term for a sociological psychology,' *Philosophy of the Social Sciences* 5: 43–62.

Weigert, Andrew (1981) *Sociology of Everyday Life*, New York: Longman.

Weinstein, George (1977) 'Natural history of retinitis pigmentosa,' in Maurice Landers, Myron Wolbarsht, John Dowling, and Alan Latics (eds) *Retinitis Pigmentosa*, New York: Plenum Press.

Williams, T. Franklin (1978) 'Diabetes mellitus in the aged,' in William Reichel (ed.) *Clinical Aspects of Aging*, Baltimore: Williams & Wilkins.

Winston, Chester (1970) 'On the realization of blindness,' *New Outlook for the Blind* 64: 16–24.

Woodruff, Diana and Birren, James (1975) *Aging: Scientific Perspectives and Social Issues*, New York: Van Nostrand.

Wrong, Dennis (1970) 'The oversocialized conception of man in modern sociology,' in Gregory Stone and Harvey Farberman (eds) *Social Psychology Through Symbolic Interactionism*, Waltham, MA: Xerox College Publishing.

Young, Pauline (1966) *Scientific Social Surveys and Research*, Englewood Cliffs, NJ: Prentice-Hall.

Index

Adams, George, 47
affiliation, 89
Aging, and body, ix–x, 54–6, 93,
120, 123; demographics of, 1,
123–4; and narrative, 94–5; and
social relationships, 92–3;
theories of, 141–7
Ainlay, Stephen, 29, 59, 136
Albert, Daniel, 19
Albrecht, R., 144
Altshuler, K., 47
Anderson, Barbara, 108
anomy, xii
Argyle, Michael, 61
Atchley, Robert, 123, 132

Back, Kurt, 46
Baldwin, Alfred, 138
Bauman, Mary, 47, 148–9
Becker, Ernest, 125–6
Becker, Gaylene, 78, 123
Becker, Howard, 128, 144
belonging identity, 77, 87
Benedek, T., 140
Bengtson, Vern, 87, 144
Berger, Peter, xii, 22, 40, 57–8,
59–60, 64, 69, 86, 88, 91, 106,
109–13, 118, 124
Bernstein, Norman, 22
Birdwhistell, Ray, 60
Blank, H. Robert, 148–9
blindness, avoidance of, 5, 37, 53–
4, 61–6, 74; commonsense
explanations of, 29;
demographics of, 9–11, 131–5;

language of, 8–19; in literature,
ix, 5; and loss, 91–5; measures
of, 8–9; stereotypes of, ix, 51–4,
66–8, 76; and stigma, 62, 122;
theories of, 147–52
body, 21; and consciousness, 22,
120–2; and identity, 20–1, 54–9,
118–27; and intentions, 24, 55–6
Bogdan, Robert, 128–9, 131
Braverman, Sydell, 148–9
Brooks, Karen, 82
Brunner, Jerome, 94
Buhler, Charlotte, 145–6
Burgess, Ernest, 22, 130–1, 144
Butler, Robert, 97, 100

cataracts, 15–16, 26, 48
Cavan, Ruth, 144
Chalkey, Thomas, 19
changing social network, 72–6
Charme, Stuart, 113–14
Chevigny, Hector, 51, 148
chronic conditions, 123
Cicourel, Aron, 129
Clark, Margaret, 108
Clausen, John, 71
coaching, 80–5
communication, difficulties with,
34, 60–4
Coni, Nicholas, 14
consumer groups, 31, 75–7, 82,
130; as alternative source of
power, 78
'consumer' vs. 'client', 85
courtesy stigma, 65

163

Index

covering, 62
Cowen, Emery, 149
crisis situation, turning points, marginal situations, 24, 106
Crosby, Faye, 29
Cumming, Elaine, 143
Curle, Adam, 77
Cutsforth, Thomas, x, 149

daily activities, difficulties with, 32–8, 55
Davis, Carl, 150
Davis, Fred, 22, 24, 67
Davis, Kingsley, 142
Dean, Janet, 61
de Beauvoir, Simone, 55–6, 73, 97, 108, 125
defensive avoidance, denial, 25, 53–4
Denzin, Norman, 128–9, 131
dependency, 71–2, 85; and powerlessness, 78
diabetic retinopathy, 17, 97–8, 99, 107
discontinuities of old age, 93
Dover, Francis, 39, 47, 50, 59
Dunn, Susan, 82
Durkheim, Emile, 138

Eden, John, 12, 15–18
Eisenstadt, S.N., 142–3
emotional syllogism, 66; see also blindness, stereotypes of
Erikson, Erik, 94–5, 99, 106, 140–1, 146–7
eye, components of, 12–19

Faraday, Annabel, 128, 129, 130
Fitzgerald, Roy, 29, 47, 49
Foner, Anne, 142
Freedman, Saul, 47
Freeman, Mark, 94
Frenkel-Brunswick, Else, 146
Freud, Sigmund, 138–41, 145–7
Friedenwald, J.S., 15

Geertz, Clifford, 106
Gergen, Kenneth, 46

glaucoma, 16–17, 27–8, 47–8, 98
Goffman, Erving, 59, 62–6, 68–9, 75, 76–9, 82, 86–8, 92, 122, 150–1
Gowman, Alan, 150
Gurwitsch, George, 39

Halasa, Adnan, 14, 16
Hall, Edward, 42
hardware, stigma symbols, 44–5 92, 107
Havighurst, Robert, 144
Helen Keller syndrome, 82
Henry, William, 143
hidden blind, 10
Husserl, Edmund, 40

'I-can-do-it-again' idealization, 40, 55
identity, xi–xii, 54–8, 79, 116–22; and aging, 118–22; and body, 20–1, 54–8, 59, 120; and social world, 77–90, 120–2; theories of, 136–41
identity-in-the-world, 59, 79, 86–90, 91, 116–18, 124–7, 136
integrity vs. despair, 94–114; as transcending individuality, 108–10; roads to, 101–8; social context of, 110–14

Jernigan, Kenneth, 31
Jervis, Frederick, 70, 79
Johnson, Marilyn, 142
Josephson, Eric, 150

Kasper, Robert, 14–18
Kaufman, Sharon, 124
Keller, Helen, 3, 6, 82
Kellner, Hansfried, 113
Kendon, Adam, 61
kinesics, 60
Kirchner, Corinne, 8–11, 132
Kirtley, Donald, 47, 148–9
Kleck, Robert, 66
Koestler, Frances, 30
Kornzweig, Abraham, 15–17
Kubler-Ross, Elisabeth, 71
Kutner, Bernard, 144

164

For Product Safety Concerns and Information please contact our EU
representative GPSR@taylorandfrancis.com
Taylor & Francis Verlag GmbH, Kaufingerstraße 24, 80331 München, Germany

www.ingramcontent.com/pod-product-compliance
Ingram Content Group UK Ltd.
Pitfield, Milton Keynes, MK11 3LW, UK
UKHW021112180425
457613UK00005B/51